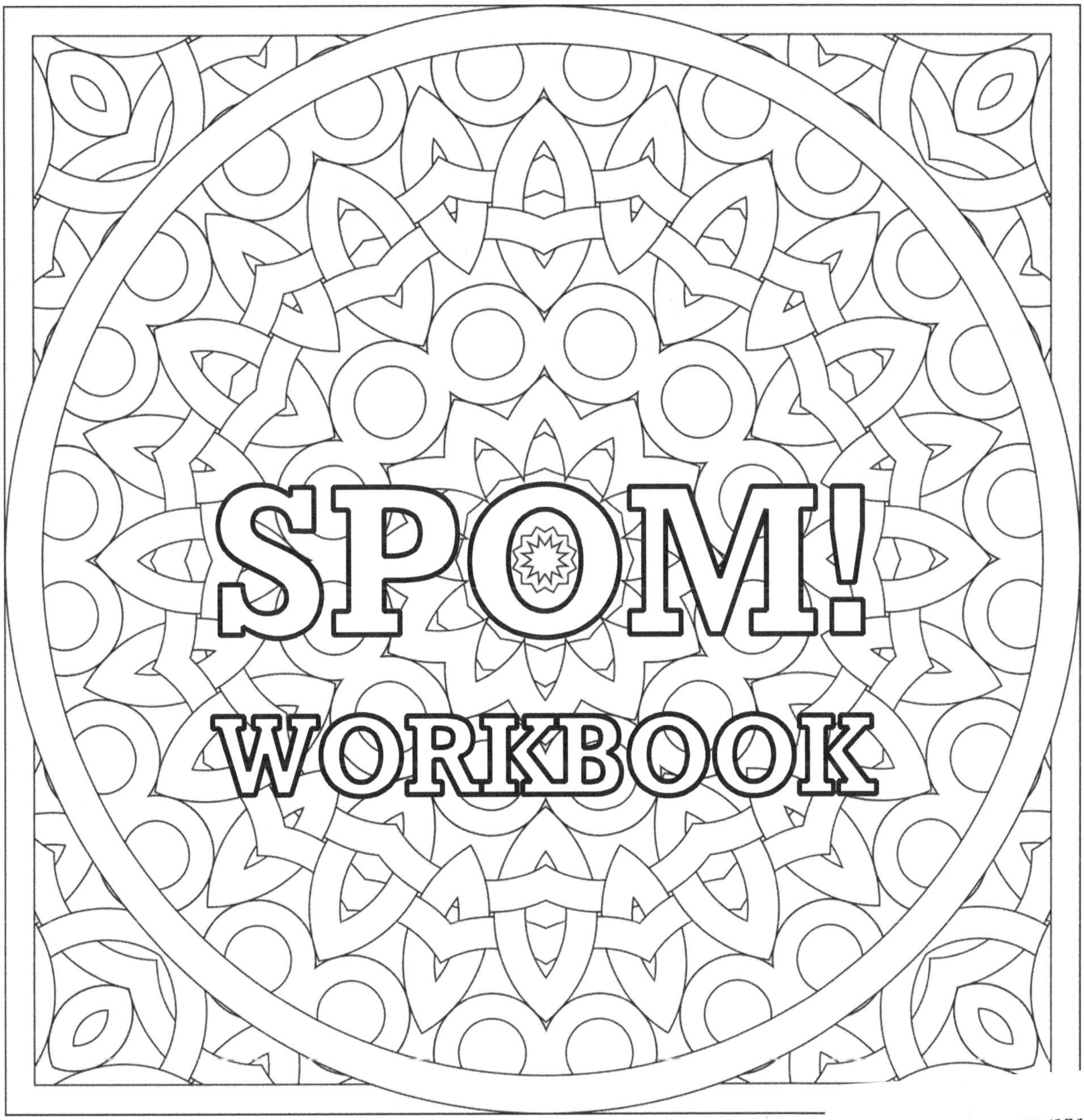

SPOM! WORKBOOK

Color Me Inspired.

The **Stop Picking On Me** *Workbook*
provides step-by-step action plans and exercises
based on the revolutionary SPOM! recovery system
for Excoriation (Skin Picking) Disorder (SPD).

DISCLAIMER: This book is sold for information purposes only. The information in this book is not intended or implied to be a substitute for professional medical advice, diagnosis or treatment either directly or indirectly, because the authors and the publishers of this work are not medical doctors. All content, including text, graphics, images and information, contained in or available here is for general information purposes only. The authors, their agents, representatives, directors and members make no representation and assume no responsibility for the accuracy of information contained on or available, and such information is subject to change. You are encouraged to confirm any information obtained from or through this book with other sources, and review all information regarding any medical condition or treatment with your physician. The intent of the author is to information is of a general entertaining nature to help you in your quest for spiritual well-being. In the event you use any of the information in this book for yourself, which is your constitutional right, neither the author nor the publisher will be held accountable and assume no responsibility for your actions, adverse effects or consequences of any kind resulting from the use or misuse of any suggestions or procedures described hereafter.

NEVER DISREGARD PROFESSIONAL MEDICAL ADVICE OR DELAY SEEKING MEDICAL TREATMENT BECAUSE OF SOMETHING YOU HAVE READ ON OR ACCESSED ONLINE OR THROUGH A BOOK.

All product and company names are trademarks™ or registered® trademarks of their respective holders. No infringement is implied. Use of them does not imply any affiliation with, disapproval of, nor endorsement by them. Products names are used as an illustrative device only.

Library of Congress Cataloging-in-Publication Data
Stratton, Mary-Margaret
SPOM! Workbook – This Workbook is designed as a companion book to the very detailed SPOM main text. It will be fun, challenging and requires your participation and it will help you stay motivated, positive and totally inspired. This highly interactive workbook takes the guesswork out of trying to figure exactly what your triggers are and encourages you to be proactive in making huge strides in your personal recovery. This book absolutely requires crayon, markers or colored pencils!

ISBN-13 978-1979643283 CreateSpace
ISBN-10: 1979643288

1. Self Help/Recovery
2. Skin Ailments
3. Compulsive Behavior
I. Stratton, Mary-Margaret II. Title

Published by Futura House
2620 South Maryland Parkway #345
Las Vegas, NV 89109
Printed in the United States of America
www.futurahouse.com

Book Design by MM Stratton (megorama.com) using GeoSlab, Times Roman and Calligraphic 421 fonts.
Please visit www.StopPickingOnMe.com
First Edition

CONTENTS

FUNDAMENTALS

ANALYSIS

DIET & PRODUCTS

ACTIONS

CONTRACTS & PRINTOUTS

NEW BEGINNINGS

ANSWERS

<u>WELCOME</u>

The ***SPOM! Workbook*** is the companion book to the official main text, ***Stop Picking On Me*** (SPOM!) text book. If you do not understand the purpose of some of the exercises in this book, the ***Stop Picking On Me*** book will help to enlighten you. It is highly recommended that you get it, because I go into very deep detail about the biological, physiological and psychological basis for this recovery program approach.

While I would like for you to go through this Workbook starting from page one and go through page by page to the end, please don't feel like you have to do that. Consider jumping around from section to section and do whatever exercise, writing, assessment, puzzle or activity that catches your eye. The point is to make sure this workbook does not become a chore, but becomes a joyous place of your self-discovery.

Have fun and please remember to color and doodle in the margins!

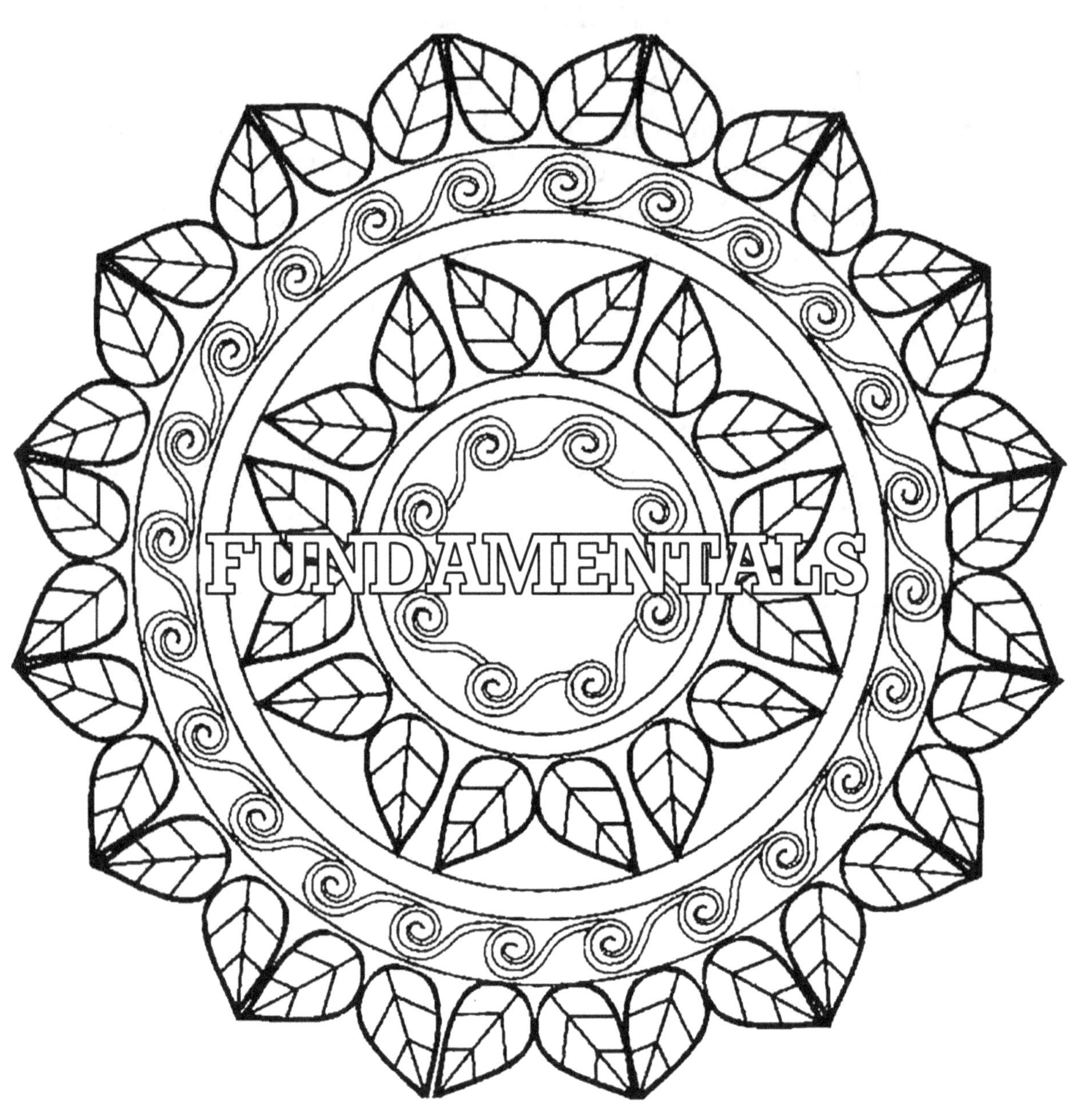

Color Me Curious.

FEELING FACES

How are you feeling right now? (Add two more!)

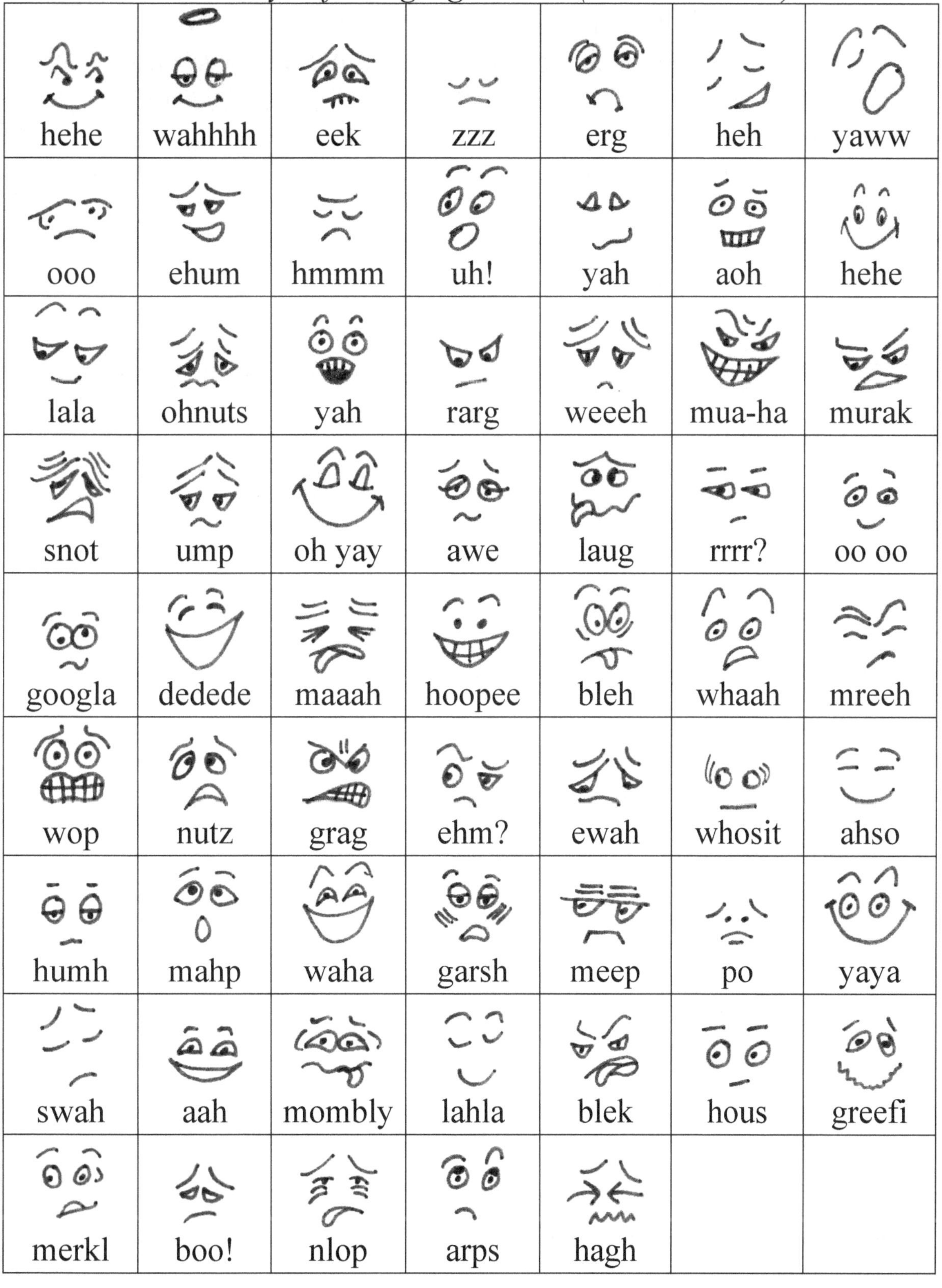

hehe	wahhhh	eek	zzz	erg	heh	yaww
ooo	ehum	hmmm	uh!	yah	aoh	hehe
lala	ohnuts	yah	rarg	weeeh	mua-ha	murak
snot	ump	oh yay	awe	laug	rrrr?	oo oo
googla	dedede	maaah	hoopee	bleh	whaah	mreeh
wop	nutz	grag	ehm?	ewah	whosit	ahso
humh	mahp	waha	garsh	meep	po	yaya
swah	aah	mombly	lahla	blek	hous	greefi
merkl	boo!	nlop	arps	hagh		

<u>TRUTH MUST BE TOLD</u>

These first two pages have no scoring system at the end. They're just to help you really get in touch with some core issues right from the start. Now I know that feelings change from day to day and even hour to hour, so just answer where you're at in an overall sense. Seeing stuff like this spelled out on paper can help bring reality to light. And sometimes self-harming people, live in a quasi-state of reality. So it's a good thing to get real!

Check out where you stand with these statements:

Statement	Agree	Maybe	Disagree
I'd do anything to avoid feeling abandoned.			
It's hard for me to concentrate.			
I don't know who I am anymore.			
It's difficult to remember the last time I felt happy.			
I often feel empty inside.			
I have problems sleeping.			
I sometimes cannot control my anger.			
I feel spaced out a lot.			
I am suspicious of others intentions.			
I feel suicidal.			
I feel worthless.			
I tend to be spontaneous to the point of being self-destructive.			

Statement	Agree	Maybe	Disagree
I cannot stop thinking about my body problems.			
I don't have a lot of stable, dependable relationships around me.			
I feel sad most of the time.			
My appetite is not what it used to be.			
I have given up hope.			
I don't get pleasure out of many things.			
I think about dying.			
I feel hopeless about my future.			
I have tried every therapy and diet and just know nothing will work.			

If you agree with the last statement above, please be willing to accept that there still might be key recovery information out there that you haven't learned yet.

If you have any checkmarks in the "agree" column, it sounds to me like you may have hit that dark bottom kind of place. What do you think? Have you had enough? In typical addiction, like alcoholism, drug addiction, or any other kind of addiction, sometimes it takes you to some pretty dark places. Sometimes you have to hit that bottom, to make the solid, never looking back, decision to get up and out of that space *for good*. Use this place of darkness as your strength. Remember it well with profound empathy and reflection, because it's never going to look like that again. And bless this day of darkness, because many people who don't ever hit that dark place, seldom get the inspiration to radically change their lives like you're going to do.

CREATE YOUR SELF-PORTRAIT

Draw a portrait of yourself the way you feel or see yourself today. You can draw yourself quite literally as a flesh and bones body, or a stick figure with callouts, or draw yourself as a cat or a cloud, or a plant or a bucket of water. There are no right or wrong ways to be creative.

Just draw!

<u>WHO AM I?</u>

Self-Definition

Do you know who you are? Really? Please answer this first question "Who am I?" Don't think about this at all, just use your name followed by any words that you would normally use to describe yourself in daily conversations, or perhaps to someone you just met. Use the first words that come to your mind. Please don't edit.

____

____

____

When you described yourself, do you describe yourself in terms of your physical characteristics, your talents, where you were from, how you relate to the world (optimistic/pessimistic), how you generally feel (happy/sad), or something else? Now that I have whet your whistle, answer the question again and be more descriptive in a deeper way:

____

____

____

____

Which of these words or phrases about yourself do you like?
Circle them.

Which would you like to change? Cross them out.

Did somebody specific in your life ever use the words you now use to describe yourself? If so, think about that person or persons for a second. How good or bad was your relationship with them? If it was anything but a stellar relationship, let their assessments of you go for now. Let's just focus on what you suspect might be the true and real positive truth about yourself.

They say that the third time is the charm. Now what words do you wish you *could* use to describe yourself? Craft the perfect self-definition of who you are way deep down inside, only focusing and featuring those traits or characteristics that you want to have around for the rest of your life. Describe yourself in terms of your childlike perfection and vast potential.

____

____

____

____

____

ADMITTANCE

Try these statements on for size and see if you can get behind saying these out loud to yourself in the mirror. Choose the first or the second feeling (in the parenthesis), whichever you relate to at the moment.

I feel (unloved / loved), and   I AM Lovable.

I feel (scared / safe), and   I AM Protected.

I feel (hopeless / hopeful), and   I AM Optimistic.

No matter how you feel in the moment, the "I AM" statement is still the same. Feeling does not ever define *who you are,* Now add a few of your own. Make up your own admittances, just remember to separate your "I AM" statements from how you feel. Feelings come and go. Get into the regular practice of never using I AM statements unless they are 100% positive about yourself. Get in the practice of using the words, "I feel."

I feel ____.

I AM____.

I feel ____.

I AM____.

I feel ____.

I AM____.

I feel ____.

I AM____.

I feel ____.

I AM____.

MY POSITIVE PERSONALITY TRAITS

Circle all that apply *(and feel free to add more)*.

Loved	Confident	Humorous	Excited
Satisfied	Thoughtful	Inspired	Serene
Grateful	Trusted	Accepted	Peaceful
Intelligent	Sensitive	Well Rested	Organized
Tenacious	Hopeful	Fascinated	Enthralled
Joyful	Playful	Loving	Happy
Willing	Courteous	Compassionate	Good listener
Trustworthy	Pleased	Honest	Spiritual
A Good Friend	Hard Working	Kind	Accepting

My Character Defects

Which 'negative' words do you identify with? Circle them. Now go through this list and cross off any character defects that you would like to release *(and feel free to add more)*.

Angry	Judgmental	Stubborn	Lazy
Hateful	Dramatic	Critical	Disorganized
Frustrated	Embarrassed	Irritable	A cry baby
Resentful	Disappointed	Ambivalent	Shameful
Shy	Exhausted	Liar	Suspicious
Weak	Ashamed	Cowardly	Outraged
Betrayed	Wishy-washy	Unsteady	Incompetent
Scared	Traumatized	Annoyed	Guilty
Irresponsible	An approval seeker	Afraid of authority	Addicted to excitement

WHERE DID I COME FROM?

Let's look at your genetic inheritance, especially the two people who lent their DNA to create this thing called you! Put down the name of your birth parents (if you know them). List your siblings (make a note if biological or adopted or step). Just jot down some basic character traits that you associate with each of these people. Make notes if you have ever witnessed or heard about any impulsive, obsessive, or compulsive behaviors for everyone on this page. Or remember if anyone had any particular sugar or carbohydrate cravings?

Birth Mother

Birth Father

Siblings

Additional Guardian Figures

Other parental-type people that figured closely in your life:
Step, Adopted or Foster Parent(s), Grandparents, Aunts or Uncles?

CHILDHOOD ABUSE TRACKER

If you suffered from any kind of childhood abuse, a professional counselor can be very helpful in healing those horrible wounds. If you say, 'it was no big deal,' without 'dealing' with what happened you are asking for psychological trouble. No human alive should have to go through childhood abuse, and it is no crime to get emotional support to figure out what happened, and why you were not to blame.

Also, it should be noted that the abuser should not be vilified. Most likely, they were abused as children themselves and were acting out of the example they were given. The cycle of repetition can and will stop with you when you go through the process of getting support.

Get the basic facts down here, but please consider creating a separate journal for processing these emotions if you do not already have one.

My age(s) _(and year(s) it happened)_

____

Abuser(s) and their role(s) in my life:

____

What happened?

____

____

Who I told or didn't tell? And what happened after that?

____

Who was blamed?

____

Why did the abuse stop?

____

CREATE A FAMILY TREE
OF DYSFUNCTION!

Now it's time to draw your family tree. You have heard the stories about that crazy aunt or drunk uncle. Put the branches and roots on your tree and include "leaf" notes about any character defects they may have exhibited. No wonder we all have issues?!?!

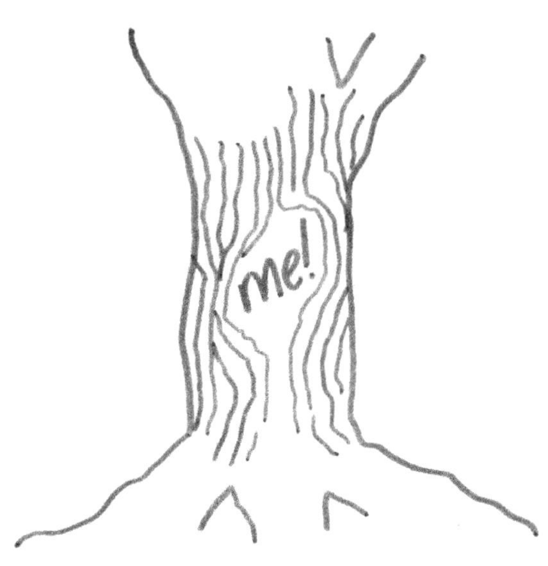

FORMATIVE YEARS

So we talked about your family background. Now I would like for you to explore significant or traumatic events/injuires/sickness that happened before you were ten-twelve years old (as early as you can remember). Explain what happened, why you think it happened, how you felt about it then, and what trait(s) you may have developed as a result of that event. Allow yourself to grieve over these events. Now that you're wiser, could you change the way you look at that formative event?

Event	Why	Feeling	Current Result
Example: My parents always argued and got divorced when I was seven.	*They married too young and always had money problems.*	*I felt like I was some kind of burden to my father. I wanted to protect mom.*	*I became very independent and refused to get involved too young myself. I distrust men.*

Event	Why	Feeling	Current Result

WHERE HAVE I BEEN?

You have probably already lived someplace. So let's get a handle on the places where you've lived. Write down the city and state. Note how old were you and the years you can remember. Make note on whether the location was urban or suburban or rural. What was the living environment like? Did you live in a single family home or an apartment? Did you have your own room or bathroom or did you have to share with people? Who else was living there? And how were they affecting your quality life – for the better or for the worse? For each place where you have lived, please answer: What did I like about living here? And what didn't I like about this place?

Where have I lived?

____

____

____

____

____

____

____

____

____

SCHOOL

Now let's look at your scholastic history. Start as early as you can remember. Try to put down dates and the name of any of your teachers. Who were your friends? How did you meet them? Why did you like those people? Did you have any enemies or people you didn't like or that just plain bugged you? Why did they affect you?

Nursery School

____

Kindergarten

____

____

Elementary School

____

____

Middle School

____

____

High School

____

____

____

College

(Or any vocational classes you have taken after high school)

____

____

____

Post College

____

____

As you look back over your school career, do you see any patterns in how you felt about your teachers? Did you have any issues with authority figures?

____

____

____

How about those friends. Do you see any patterns about the kinds of people you hung out with? If you could do it all over again, would you choose the same types of people? Why or why not?

____

____

____

WONDERFUL WORD FIND

Take a break from the hard thinking work and have fun with this puzzle!

Answers on Page 129

B	B	L	E	S	S	M	E	L	B	A	V	O	L	T
L	F	E	E	L	M	L	A	O	A	P	P	L	E	L
E	L	F	A	F	A	L	P	V	R	A	R	B	G	M
S	M	A	R	U	R	A	D	A	T	H	E	M	O	C
S	P	R	E	T	T	Y	M	I	L	F	A	H	A	E
E	T	R	E	E	R	I	E	G	R	I	F	P	L	Y
D	C	R	L	A	Y	N	F	E	I	T	A	A	P	I
L	A	O	A	R	T	H	E	U	C	B	B	P	E	T
U	T	C	M	G	N	I	V	O	L	F	A	P	A	N
F	I	A	A	P	E	M	P	E	M	H	C	S	C	A
E	N	L	R	R	E	H	A	N	D	S	O	M	E	I
T	I	M	P	O	R	T	A	N	T	S	T	A	F	D
A	F	G	N	I	L	A	E	H	H	A	N	R	U	A
R	M	L	A	T	T	A	I	N	G	O	A	L	L	R
G	R	A	T	E	S	T	R	A	T	E	G	I	E	S

Words to find:

- AttainGoal
- Beautiful
- BeFree
- Blessed
- Calm
- Capable
- Competent
- Grateful
- Handsome
- Happy
- Healing
- Important
- Lovable
- Loving
- Patient
- Peaceful
- Pretty
- Radiant
- Smart
- Strategies

My History

Basics

I was born in *(Year)* ________________________________

I started to become aware of my body and skin changing around:

(Year and age) _______________________________________

I noticed feeling "imperfect" in some way in around:

(Year and age) _______________________________________

This was right around the time that:

(What was happening) _________________________________

____

The types of breakout I typically get are:

Blackhead   Whitehead   Pimple   Pustule   Nodule   Cyst   Scar

They appear on my:

Chin   Neck   Forehead   Nose   My face

Back   Legs   Behind   Chest   Other

My acne started out being:

Mild   Moderate   Severe

Since that time, my acne has become:

More severe   Less severe   About the same

The impact of this condition makes my life:

Acceptable   Difficult   Unbearable

Lifestyle and Habits

I typically sleep

Less than 7 hours	7-9 hours	More than 9 hours

I generally sleep

Lightly	Soundly	With Issues

I drink or smoke a substance to relax me

Daily	Few Times a Week	Weekly
Monthly	Socially	Rarely or Never

I use coffee, tea, energy drinks or other substances to keep me going

Daily	Few Times a Week	Weekly
Monthly	Socially	Rarely or Never

I take something to help me with pain

Daily	Few Times a Week	Weekly
Monthly	Socially	Rarely or Never

I get myself moving with some kind of (mild or strenuous) exercise

Daily	Few Times a Week	Weekly
Monthly	Socially	Rarely or Never

I started my first job at: *(Year and age)* _______________________

Working made me feel:

____

Women: My monthly cycles tend to last *(Days)* _______________________

Women: My monthly cycles

are regular	are irregular and sometimes painful	just miserable
filled with bloating	make me moody	initiate breakout madness

Medications and Supplements

I am on the following pharmaceutical medications:

____

____

____

The side effects listed for these medications include:

____

____

____

____

I take the following supplements:

____

____

____

The side effects listed for these supplements include:

____

____

Besides the side effects listed above, women please take a close look at
your hormones and if there are issues, bring this up with a good doctor.
Also consider what substances you are using to get yourself through the
week. Could these be adding toxins and affecting you adversely?

WHERE AM I GOING?

When you were very little you probably daydreamed about doing something in particular when you grew up. Now we all can't be president of the United States or a big movie star, but see if you can see beyond those limited childlike ambitions and narrow it to something like, I liked and wanted to be a leader or I like and wanted to entertain people and make them happy.

These goals are totally achievable and you can make a big difference in the world without even being President!

Occupation

Describe your dream job(s), career(s) or occupation(s) in vivid detail. If you don't know what that is, at least list the things that you would enjoy doing regardless whether or not you were getting paid.

What are the qualities you list on Page 14 and the top of 16 that would make you good at this activity? And what qualities (if any) will you have to develop to attract that dream pasttime?

RELATIONSHIPS

What is your ideal relationship scenario?

____

____

Is this person currently in your life or have you met them before at some point?

1) If they are in your life now, describe how that relationship status is going compared to your ideal relationship scenario.

2) If you have met them before, are they still in your life? And if they are not, can you describe what happened? Why are they not currently in your life?

3) If you have not met this person(s) yet, do you believe that you will? Why or why not?

____

____

____

____

LEGACY

At the end of your life, how do you want to remembered? I know this may sound morbid, but please write your own obituary. Fantasize about the kind of life you intend to live in the future and write your obit as if you were living an idealized life. Describe what you contributed to your community. Who are you survived by?

WHY NOT PICK?

I am sure you have taken a lot of time trying to figure WHY you do what you do. I used to ask myself that question for years and years. But have you ever wondered the opposite. What will you gain from NOT picking. See which statements are reasons NOT to pick.

Statement	Agree	Maybe	Disagree
When I pick I get upset with myself.			
I scare the people who care about me.			
I don't spend time/effort on empowering myself in other better long-lasting ways.			
I have problems at work.			
I might kill myself accidentally.			
I feel like a loser.			
I might have to be hospitalized for mental illness.			
Picking has its own mind and will over my mind and will.			
People will think I have no self-control.			
I have problems at school.			
I might scar myself accidentally.			
I have problems in my relationship(s).			

Can you add any more reasons to stop this insanity? Because you can do it. So gather up your reasons why you'll chose not to pick anymore.

PERFECTION OBSERVATION

In the main SPOM! Text, I suggest an exercise where you go out into a beautiful natural setting and observe as many imperfections as you can. Write down your observations of all the gooey, sticky, messy, rough, missing pieces and chewed up things you see naturally occurring in nature. Then take time to reflect on how you can allow this to change the way you feel about yourself.

MEDITATION - FLAME OF ATTENTION

Now that you have put some thought into defining who you are, where you come from and where you are going, please take a minimum fifteen minute break to ponder what you may have recently uncovered.

Light a candle and just sit and stare at the flame. Just sit quietly with your thoughts. Reflect on any 'aha' moments you might have had. Has it been a while since you thought about that drunk uncle? Are you surprised at the self-definition words that came up that you now want to cross off your list? Have you taken time to think about that place you once lived in and how it made you feel to be there? This is a meditation where it's okay to let your mind wander. Allow yourself to see if any other memories pop up, or anything else comes to mind.

If that happens, make sure you record those thoughts here, because they may be useful in your future recovery.

____

____

____

____

____

____

____

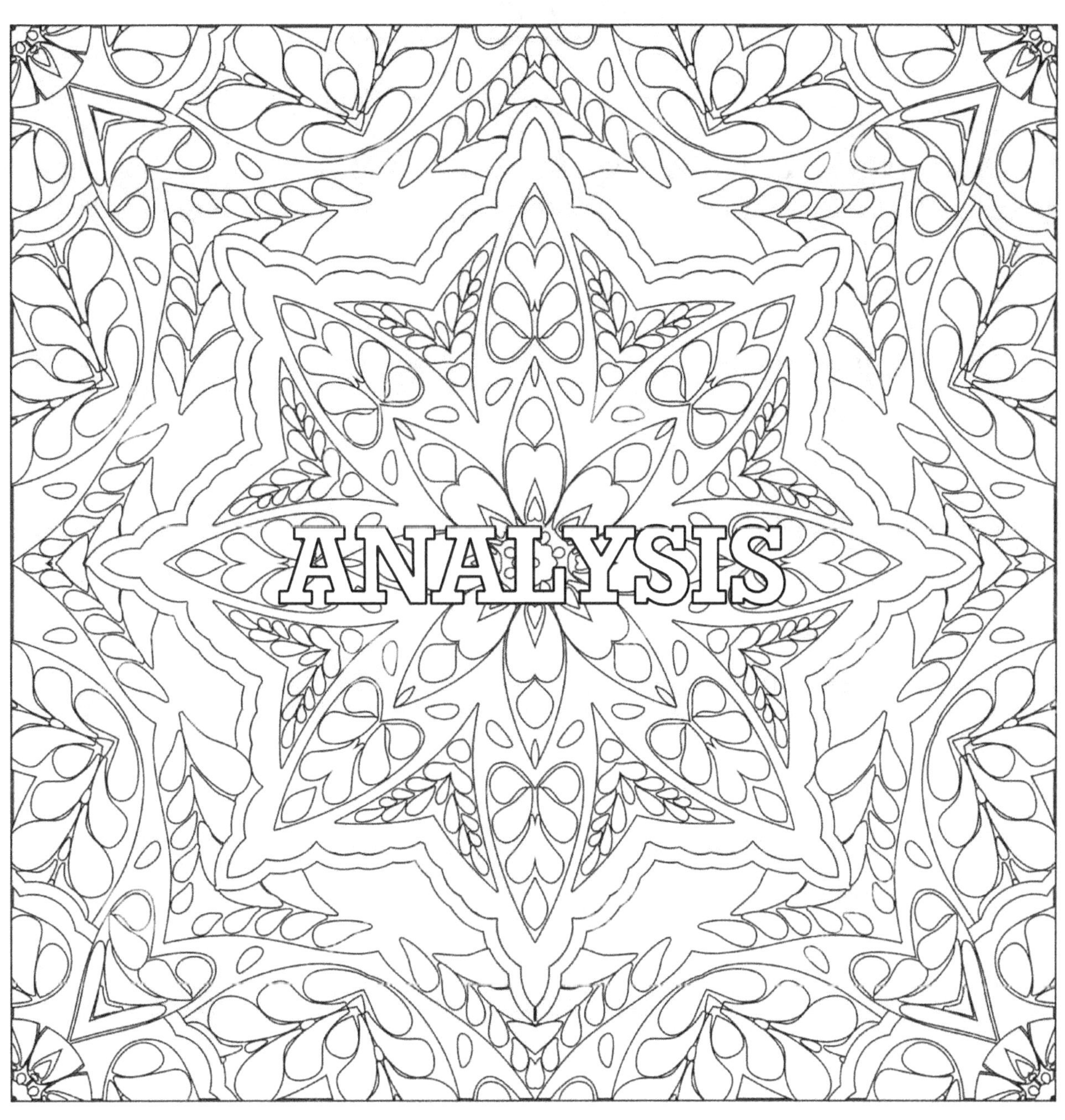

Color Me Intelligent.

21 QUESTIONS

(adapted from the <u>Kiss Addiction Goodbye</u> Book)

Circle every one you answer "yes" to. Count how many "yes" answers you have. Then turn the page and see how you did on this stress test.

1. I smoke (tobacco or any herb).
2. I worry about money.
3. I suffer from chronic pain.
4. I have been divorced.
5. I am not in a happy relationship.
6. I need more exercise.
7. I have trouble sleeping.
8. I have constipation issues.
9. I am long overdue for a vacation.
10. I get tension headaches.
11. My family is dysfunctional.
12. I have a few too many extra pounds.
13. I skip meals to get the job done.
14. I eat foods impulsively just because they sound good to me in the moment.
15. My stomach has 'issues' after eating.
16. I have usually have a daily glass of wine, beer or cocktail.
17. Sex? What's that?
18. I eat out a lot.
19. I wish I could get a better job.
20. I take meds for depression.
21. I feel chronically overwhelmed, wiped out, and wish I had more time.

How many "yes" answers did you get?

Less than 5 = Low Stress
Time to write a book and share what you are doing right!

5-10 = Moderate Stress
You could probably use this book!
But don't stress on it!

More than 10 = High Stress
You really really need this book!
But don't stress on it!

More than 15 = Very High Stress
Read this book tonight, and don't put it down until you're done!
But seriously, don't stress on it!

Tracking your patterns

The next couple of exercises will help you start to track where your
'danger' zones are. This is really important, because if you tend to self-
harm in the evening (like I used to), then you know that is when you
have to be on extra alert to catch yourself from stumbling. And it means
that you will have to have some good strategies in place to help you
through those especially difficult time periods.

ASSOCIATIONS

Think about the first things that come to mind to fill in the rest of these statements. Are your associations positive or negative or a combination of both? Write and simply observe your reactions.

My face is…

My skin is…

My body is…

My health is…

My spirit is…

My soul is…

Movie star or 'celebrity' faces are…

Movie star or 'celebrity' skin is…

Movie star or 'celebrity' bodies are…

Habit Assessment Chart

Make some serious notes about your behavior for a whole day. Please don't do this on a day off. You probably don't get many of those and I would like to see you use those to completely forget about picking altogether and do some other fun activity. Try to track your behavior over a twenty-four hour period of time. (Include how your sleep habits fit in a normal day.)

Rate your thoughts on a scale of 1-10 on how strongly you feel urges, how often you premeditated or planned to pick, how often you succumbed to those urges, and finally how much you were able to persevere and triumph over your urges or planning.

Time	Urges	Planning	Breakdown	Success
6-8 AM				
8-10 AM				
10-Noon				
Noon-2 PM				
2-4 PM				
4-6 PM				
6-8 PM				
8-10 PM				
10-MID				
MID-2 AM				
2 -4 AM				
4-6 AM				

HABIT DIARY WEEK

Now that you have analyzed a typical day, take a week (start on any day – it does not have to be Monday) and make notes on what happened to you throughout that week. Try to do this daily and preferably keep this page with you and then put tic marks each and every time you encounter these scenarios. The idea is to become conscious of your behavior. Obviously you know *that* you do it, but do you know exactly how much and how often? And are you tracking just how much emotional distress you are encountering on a daily basis?

Day	How many times I felt anxiety or distress?	How many urges had vs actual self-harm times	Strategies used? Triggers? Observations? Feelings before/after?
Mon.			
Tues.			
Wed.			
Thur.			
Fri,			
Sat.			
Sun.			

<u>BREAKOUT JOURNAL</u>

Try to track where exactly you are finding your breaking out. Is it on your body, your face, your arms, or elsewhere? Describe the type of breakout you are finding, blackheads, pimples, rough bumpy, full blown pimples, or big cysts. Try to track these breakouts for a few days in a row. Remember sometimes where you break out and how you breakout may give you a clue to other internal issues that you can bring up with your doctor.

Time of Day	Location	Type of Congestion
Morning		
Noon		
Evening		
Night		
Morning		
Noon		
Evening		
Night		
Morning		
Noon		
Evening		
Night		

Create Modern Art - How Does it Feel?

Now that you have put down *analytically* what you have been doing on paper, how do you feel about self-harming behavior? Can you draw the feeling? (Remember the feeling is NOT your self-definition – it's just the state you are in in any particular moment of time.) Use as much or as little color as you feel necessary. Does it feel like a round complete feeling? Or does it feel all rigid and squared off? Perhaps it feels all jagged? Is it cloudy gray or red hot and black? Do not attempt to draw actual 'objects,' unless you feel so strongly inclined.

Allow yourself to be an abstract Modern artist!

ACCEPTANCE AND ACTION
TYPE OF QUESTIONNAIRE

Look over the following statements and see how true they ring for you.
Then please share them with a caring doctor.

Use a scale of 1 to 5 with 1 being never true and 5 being always true.

Statement	Rating
I feel my life is not what it could be because I have had so many painful experiences and memories.	
My feelings scare me.	
I am afraid I cannot keep control of my feelings and worries.	
My life is not fulfilled due to my past experiences.	
My life is ruined by my emotions.	
I seem to be the only one I know who cannot control the quality of their life.	
I will never be successful because I worry too much.	
Total Score	

An average score might be around ten to twelve points. While someone in distress might score sixteen or higher points.

An official questionnaire similar to this was developed by Bond, F. W., S. C. Hayes, et al.in 2011. "Preliminary psychometric properties of the Acceptance and Action Questionnaire–II: A revised measure of psychological inflexibility and experiential avoidance." Behavior Therapy 42(4): 676-688.

STRESS ASSESSMENTS

(adapted from the <u>Kiss Addiction Goodbye</u> Book)

The next few pages will help you review what specific kind of stresses you have been under recently, in the last few years, or over a lifetime. You will look at

- Emotional Stress

- Cognitive Stress

- Structural Stress

- Metabolic Stress and

- Environmental Stress.

Fill out these forms on a scale of 0-10

0 =not stressful
10 being very stressful

Acknowledge what you have experienced over a lifetime, in the past two years, in the past three months, and as recent as today.

Fill everything out to the best of your ability. If you have a suspicion that an issue may go deeper, by all means, please talk to your doctor and get any tests done that will sort out the puzzle pieces for you.

Take a close look at where you see higher numbers both in the past and in your present circumstances. Have you thought about the connection between your habits and skin health and these stressors before? Are there stressful elements in your life that you have the power to change? Focus on what you have control over.

*G*D grant me the Serenity to accept the things I cannot change,*
The Courage to change the things I can,
And the Wisdom to know the difference.

Twelve Step Serenity Prayer

EMOTIONAL STRESS
(ISSUES THAT CAN CONTRIBUTE TO ANXIETY)

State	Past Day	3 months	2 years	Lifetime
Sense of Loss				
Death in Family				
PTSD				
Divorce				
Change in Job/Career				
Unhappy Job				
Weak Father				
Lack of Purpose				
No Higher Power				
Dominant Mother				
Addict in Family				
Chronic Relapse				
Relationship Issues				
Children Issues				
Non-Stop To-Do				
No Downtime				
Other (describe)				

COGNITIVE STRESS
(HOW YOU SEE YOURSELF IN THE WORLD)

State	Past Day	3 months	2 years	Lifetime
Irrational Thinking				
High Expectations				
Victim Consciousness				
Blaming Others				
Blaming Outside Circumstances				
Angry at World Issues/Figures				
Lack of Gratitude				
Living in the Past				
Living in Future				
Lack of Empathy				
Poor Memory				
Feeling Failure				
Chronic Pain (Real or Phantom)				
Other (describe)				

STRUCTURAL STRESS
(PHYSICAL ISSUES, INJURIES AND ABNORMALITIES)

State	Past Day	3 months	2 years	Lifetime
Major Injuries				
Cancer				
Joint Issues				
Postural Physical Abnormalities or Obstructions				
Flexibility Issues				
Sinus Issues				
Skin Disorders				
Parasites				
Candida				
Dental Issues				
Chronic Infections				
Bone Density Issues				
Coronary/Arterial Blockages				
Emphysema				
Sleep Apnea				
Other (describe)				

METABOLIC STRESS
(INTERNAL ISSUES. ASK YOUR DOCTOR!)

State	Past Day	3 months	2 years	Lifetime
Hormonal Changes				
Pre-Menstural Syndrome (PMS)				
Blood Sugar Imbalance (Hypo or Hyperglycemia)				
Diabetes				
Methylation Deficiencies				
Andropause				
Menopause				
Endocrine Issues				
Neurotransmitter Imbalance				
Allergies				
Autoimmune Issues				
Inflammatory Responses				
Other (describe)				

Environmental Stress (External issues)

State	Past Day	3 months	2 years	Lifetime
Mercury Toxicity				
Heavy Metals Exposure				
Food Additive Exposure				
TransFats Exposure				
Herba-Pesti-cides				
Nano Bacteria Exposure				
Molds or Fungus Exposure				
Petrochemical Exposure				
Microwave Use				
Cell Phone Use				
Relocation				
Constant Travel				
Electromagnetic Exposure				
Financial Issues				
Housing Issues				
Other (describe)				

Double Stress Scramble

Answers on Page 129

What are some possible sources of stress?

What will set you free from stress?

Unscramble the first sets of words for some answers to the first question. Then use the letters in the highlighted circles to unscramble the answer to the second question.

RCIODVE

ESABU

SEILPRANG

NPIA

XIFODOTCO

TILUG

Letters from the highlighted circles:

Unscramble those letters to find the answer:

EMOTIONAL COMPONENTS

Describe how these specific emotions affect you physically. Then describe how you cope with the feeling. Lastly admit whether your particular coping strategies to deal with these emotions works or not?

Fear

How it feels:

How I cope:

Does it work?

What else could I do?

Sadness

How it feels:

How I cope:

Does it work?

What else could I do?

Resentment

How it feels:

How I cope:

Does it work?

What else could I do?

Anger

How it feels:

How I cope:

Does it work?

What else could I do?

Frustration

How it feels:

How I cope:

Does it work?

What else could I do?

Guilt

How it feels:

How I cope:

Does it work?

What else could I do?

Shame

How it feels:

How I cope:

Does it work?

What else could I do?

PREOCCUPATION CHART

This chart will help you realize where your focus in life is and where there might be opportunity to adjust that focus. You know what they say: "What you Think About Expands." So when you obsess on your skin problems, guess what seems to never go away? And if you start to think about a life completely disconnected to bad skin and picking, guess what will expand? Check the column that matches your obsession level.

Statement	Hourly	Daily	Weekly	Rarely
I think about my skin problems.				
I must take care of the problems personally and directly.				
I feel agitated when I cannot get to my skin to check in.				
I hurt myself worse than intended.				
I have tried to quit cold turkey.				
I try to stop myself.				
I plan for the next moment I can deal with my skin.				
I think about what tools I might use to work on my skin.				
I am always looking for articles or posts on helping my skin.				
I have hurt myself without realizing how or when I did it.				
I feel my skin crawling.				

WHAT'S YOUR FOCUS?

Where are you focusing your time, energy and attention? Think about your life. Are you so preoccupied with your skin that other more important goals and plans stay in the dark?

Fill in what is in your spotlight. Then fill in everything else that is important to you that outside of the sweet spot that is *not* getting the light of your focus.

You know that have the power to move that light elsewhere.

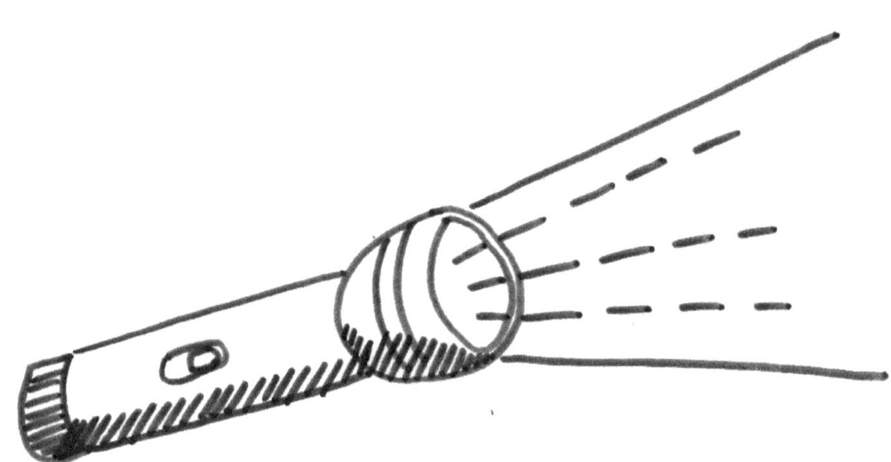

CONSEQUENCE CHARTS

Let's put picking aside for a second. Make a list of ALL the bad habits you have (everything except picking – like not exercising, drugs, eating badly, lying, spending, cheating, temper, irresponsible sex, media abuse, smoking, drinking, etc.) and write down the consequences of your actions (or inactions). Remember that self-harm (and most other 'bad' habits) usually have benefits or we would not do them. It's easy to list the not-so-good results of bad habits, but work really hard to see the good results you get out. These are some good questions to ask yourself:

- Do I feel calmer? More relaxed?

- Do I get a rush?

- Do people give me more attention or support?

- Do people leave me alone?

- Does it feel like a comfortable activity?

- Do I feel vindicated?

- Does it help protect me in some way?

- Do I feel 'excited' when I know I'm going to "do" my habit?'

- Does the habit make me feel stronger somehow?

- Docs thc habit distract me from other pressing matters?

- Does the habit communicate something to others around me that I am unable to put into actual spoken words?

- Do I expect to feel better afterwards?

- Does my mind or brain feel more 'clear' afterwards?

- Does the habit make me feel connected to my body? Or to the present moment?

Don't be afraid to see what you are getting out of these behaviors and see that it is a way you have previously coped with stress or anxiety. Now you are just learning new ways!

HOW DO BAD HABITS AFFECT YOU?

Copy this page if you need more room to list more bad habits.

Habit	Good Results	Not So Good Results

CONSEQUENCES

Now just focus only on self-harming behavior. Remember it's just another bad habit caused by physiological and psychological coping conditions. Ponder the same questions you have asked about your other bad habits, but specifically associate them with your skin and how they affect you both in short term and long term.

How it affects me in the:	Positive Results	Negative Results
Short run	*Example:* *Makes me feel in control*	*Example:* *Leaves a scab*
Long haul	*Example:* *Helps me cope with other more difficult issues*	*Example:* *Long lasting scars*

SELF-TALK

This exercise takes you being committed to being highly creative. It means you must imagine you having a talk with yourself. If you have read the SPOM book then you have two examples of how this is done.

Below are example questions you might ask yourself. Remember to write down the very first thing that pops into your mind. No editing allowed. It has to come out spontaneously. If you feel stunted or stagnant in answering, imagine that there is a person who looks exactly like you standing or sitting there staring at you waiting for you to say something. They are looking at you like, "Well, are you going to talk or not???" Put the pressure on to have a real and engaging conversation.

Especially consider asking yourself open ended questions, not just things that require a yes or no answer. Feel free to contradict yourself and even argue with yourself gently. The goal of this exercise is to get a legitimate agreement with yourself to change up your habits.

Here are some potential questions to ask yourself.

- Do you feel safe? Why or why not?

- What are you worried about?

- How willing are you to change the ending of your story?

- Tell me what makes you tick?

- Is there a strategy that you wish I would do more of?

- What is scaring you right now?

- What do you need from me?

Feel free to get extra paper in case there's not enough space to finish the entire conversation in this workbook.

My Self Talk

MIRRORING AND PARAPHRASING

Now that you have hopefully found some interesting answers about what is going on inside of you, write down a summary of what you just downloaded.

____

____

____

____

Now "mirror" yourself. Re-write what you just wrote above, but in a different way. In other words, write what you said, but use different words or phrases or language. Try this technique in other areas of your life. Sometimes trying to explain the same thing in a different way with different words allows us to get insight into thoughts or feelings we didn't recognize before.

____

____

____

____

<u>RESENTMENTS</u>

Everyone has resentments, at least until they reach Christ Consciousness or Buddha Nirvana… Until then, it's critical to get these divisive and corrosive thoughts out in the open so they can get the fresh air needed to blow them away. Look into the deeper cause of why these issues exist.

Resentment	Why this exists	How I Feel	Different Take
Example: My boss never acknowledges my contributions.	*He's probably overwhelmed with responsibility and never learned to be a graceful person.*	*Like I don't matter. I'm not important. I do good work and am ignored. I'm scared I could get laid off.*	*I know I do good work. I'll stop looking to others to validate me. Even if they don't say it, I know I'm needed.*

Resentment	Why this exists	How I Feel	Different Take

PURGE THE URGE

Urges may not magically disappear overnight. They will ebb and flow as you get healthier. You must learn to accept the urges when they arrive and let them wash over you like a wave. If you have ever swum in the ocean and you see a big wave coming, hopefully you have been taught that you hold your breath and jump straight into it. When you do that, you end up on the other side of the wave floating. And if you don't do jump through the wave, you could end up getting tumbled pretty harshly by the wave. Self-harming urges are just like that. You have to face it head on and jump through it to get to the other side of peace. On that front, it might help if you describe what an urge feels like so you can identify them and become aware the crashing wave is coming!

First, can I accept the fact that I have urges to harm myself?

____

These urges feel like:

____

If I don't yield to the urge, I will feel:

____

____

My urges usually last:

____

If I could learn to not surrender to the urge(s), I might be able to feel:

____

____

WHAT'S WORKING?

Everyone is different. Everyone heals in different ways with different timing. Go through the suggestions offered to you in the SPOM text that appealed to you and keep track of the various techniques that work best.

Sensory Distraction	What didn't work	What did work (do more of this)
• Sight		
• Sound		
• Scent		
• Touch		
• Taste		
Physical Activity		
• Exercise		
• Other Activities		
Fun Distractions		
• Playtime/Games		
• Other fun things		
Mindful Practices		
• Relaxation Techniques		
• Yoga/ Meditation		
• Writing/journaling		
• Other Mindfulness		

MEDITATION - I AM CONSCIOUSNESS

Take a moment to be quiet with yourself. How does it feel to be so incredibly analytical and write down all these things? Be with those feelings and name them. Does it make you feel powerless over your problems? Or does it make you feel in more control? Focus on the latter response. Try a few minutes of sitting still and breathing in and out with a series of three affirmations. You may say the words out loud, whisper them, or simply picture them in your mind's eye.

1) With your inhale, think the words, "I AM."
   And with your exhale, think the words, "uncovering."

2) With your inhale, think the words, "I AM."
   And with your exhale, think the words, "healing."

3) With your inhale, think the words, "I AM."
   And with your exhale, think the words, "in charge."

Continue to breath and repeat these three affirmations for as long as it takes for you to really accept these words as truth deep down inside your heart and soul.

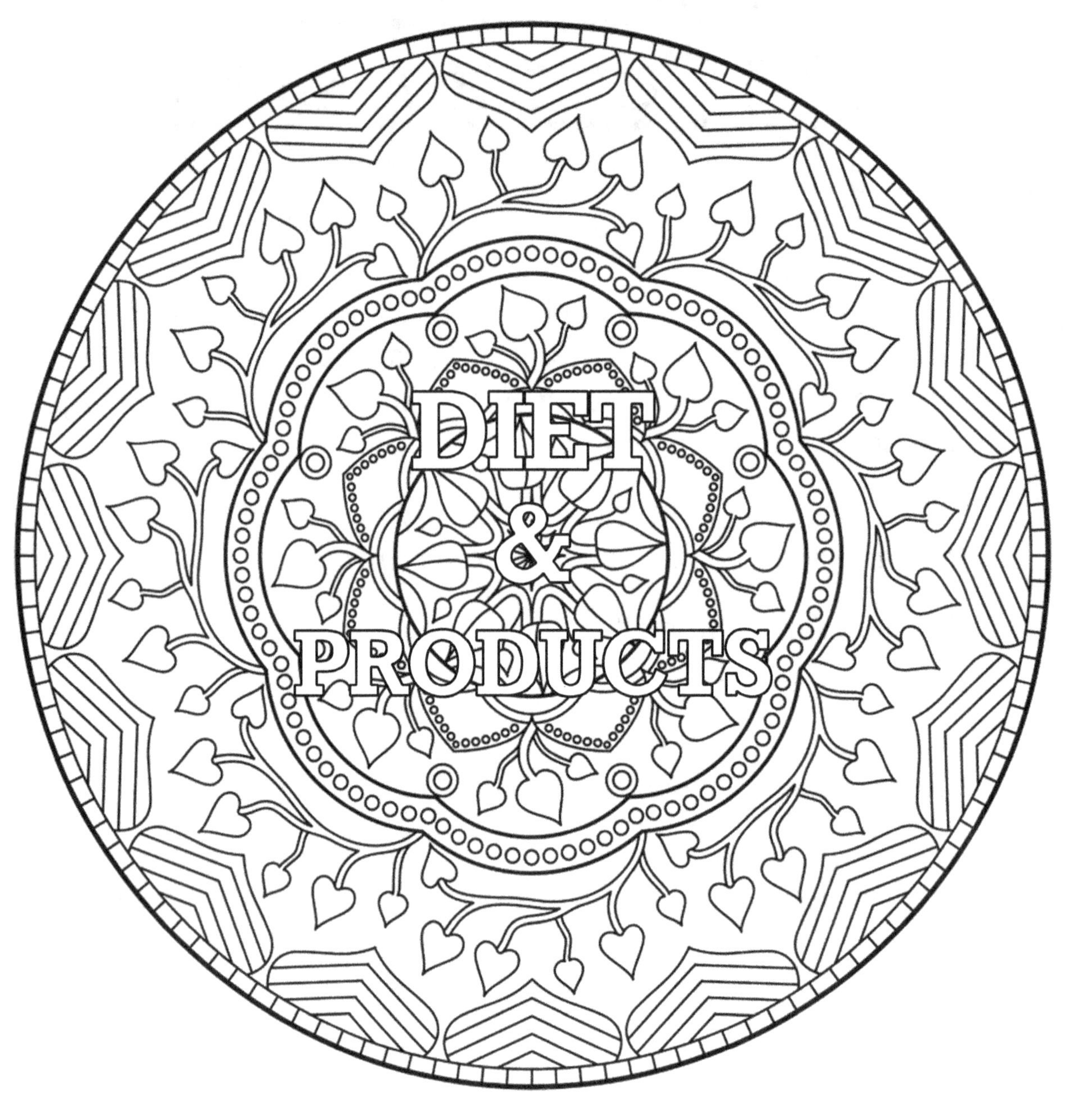

Color Me Motivated.

My Nutrition

This next section is crucial. If you have read *Stop Picking On Me* or are at least familiar with the SPOM! Program, then you know just how crucial your food intake is to get your healthy again.

Favorite Foods and Snacks

Write down a list of a few of the current foods you usually have around. List the things you tend to stock up on from the market, or the things you usually grab and go from the mini mart or fast food joint when you're in a hurry. Separate them into the columns on whether you think they are healthy for you, or not so healthy for you. No judgements allowed. Just observations here!

Healthy Foods	Not So Healthy Foods

Let's look at the not so healthy column. If your higher self knows that these food might not be your highest choice, why do you suppose you choose them? Jot down a couple of your excuses for eating them. There is no judgement here, just a desire to get to the bottom of why you do the things you do.

____

____

____

____

Now let's look at the healthy column of foods and snacks. How do you feel about yourself knowing that you have chosen to have these foods in your life. Does it make you feel good about yourself? Why do you suppose you don't eat more of them?

____

____

____

Hey! What is your favorite fruit? Please draw a picture of it!

Wasn't that fun?

THREE DAY FOOD ANALYSIS

(adapted from the Kiss Addiction Goodbye Book)

What is your diet doing for you? And where is it leading you into that muddy ugly, stuck in the problem feeling? The ultimate goal here is to eventually determine what kind of nutritional value your food intake has been providing for you. Have you been getting enough protein, fat, carbohydrate, fiber, water, vitamins or minerals? Have you been getting enough calories? A trained dietician can give you the exact details on this stuff, but for now, know that you are smart enough to take a decent non-professional overview, and be able to recognize areas for improvement, *if you just start paying attention to what you have been eating*.

Please complete a Diet Diary for three consecutive days with one day being a weekend day. Please try to give *detailed* information. And remember to include any supplements you are taking.

Food Diary Instructions

- Record information as soon as possible after the food has been consumed.

- The purpose of this food record is to analyze your *current eating habits*. This is **NOT** a test of your moral fiber or your will power or discipline. Do not change your eating behavior at this time, unless it is advised by a health practitioner.

- Describe the food or beverage consumed. e.g., milk - what kind? (Soy, almond, whole, 2%, or nonfat, etc.); toast - (whole wheat, white, buttered); chicken - (fried, baked, breaded); pizza (size of pizza, how many slices, toppings), etc.

- As closely as possible, estimate *quantity* of your portions. Record the amount of each food consumed using standard measurements as much as possible, such as approximately 8 ounces, 1/2 cup, 1 teaspoon, 3 tablespoons, 4 packets, 3 slices, etc. in your meal.

- Include any added items. For example: tea with 1 teaspoon sugar, potato with 2 teaspoons butter, etc.

- Please record all beverages and their amounts, including water. List them in a "Beverage" category.

- Record any exercise you get each day, including the type of activity and its duration. If you did any strenuous exercise, it might be good to make a note of how strenuous it was… because this could affect your dietary choices and patterns.

- Please record all bowel movements and their consistency (regular, loose, firm, etc.).

- Please also record anytime you get a specific craving. I.E. "3:40 PM had a craving for a jelly donut…"

- Note any changes in your general outlook throughout the three day period in the "Symptoms and Feelings" area of the diary. Give physical as well as emotional symptoms (e.g., bloated, tired, energetic, craving more food, irritable, etc.). Note any mood shifts through the day.

- Please write legibly enough that you can read your own writing at a later time. And if you are up to it, it would be beneficial to share this with a registered dietician or licensed nutritionist.

Do this for at least three (3) consecutive days. These food diaries are not meant to make you feel you guilty, but to start to get you aware of what you are putting in your mouth. And eventually, you may wish to go back to your various Habit and Stress Assessments and Breakout Journal along with your Initial History and regular use of substances (look at anything you wrote on Page 27) and see if there are any noticeable connections?

FOOD DIARY EXAMPLE

Not Enough Detail

Breakfast:

- pancakes
- eggs
- bacon
- juice
- coffee

Lunch:

- chicken burrito
- diet coke

Snack:

- crackers
- handful of nuts
- cheese

Better Level of Detail

Breakfast:

- 2 4-inch pancakes w/ ¼ cup syrup
- 2 scrambled eggs
- 2 slices turkey bacon
- 1 tablespoon margarine

Beverages:

- 6 oz. fresh orange juice
- 2 cups coffee w/2 packets NutraSweet™
- ¼ cup half and half

Lunch:

- 1 large flour tortilla
- ½ cup rice
- ½ cup black beans
- ¼ cup jack cheese
- 2 ounces chicken
- ¼ cup tomato salsa

Beverages:

- 2 diet cokes (12 oz. cans)

Snack:

- 10 wheat crackers
- ¼ cup raw almonds
- 1 oz. cheddar cheese

DAY 1_______________ **~ Date**_______________________________

Time	Foods Eaten /Amount	How Do You Feel?*
	Breakfast:	
	Morning Snack:	
	Lunch:	
	Afternoon Snack:	
	Dinner:	
	Evening Snack:	
	Exercise: Time spent +Type	
	Bowel Movements: Time/Consistency	

DAY 2_______________ **~ Date**____________________________

Time	Foods Eaten /Amount	How Do You Feel?*
	Breakfast:	
	Morning Snack:	
	Lunch:	
	Afternoon Snack:	
	Dinner:	
	Evening Snack:	
	Exercise: Time spent +Type	
	Bowel Movements: Time/Consistency	

DAY 3_________________ **~ Date**______________________________

Time	Foods Eaten /Amount	How Do You Feel?*
	Breakfast:	
	Morning Snack:	
	Lunch:	
	Afternoon Snack:	
	Dinner:	
	Evening Snack:	
	Exercise: Time spent +Type	
	Bowel Movements: Time/Consistency	

FOOD FUN CROSSWORD

Take a break and see what you can learn from this crossword.

Answers on Page 130

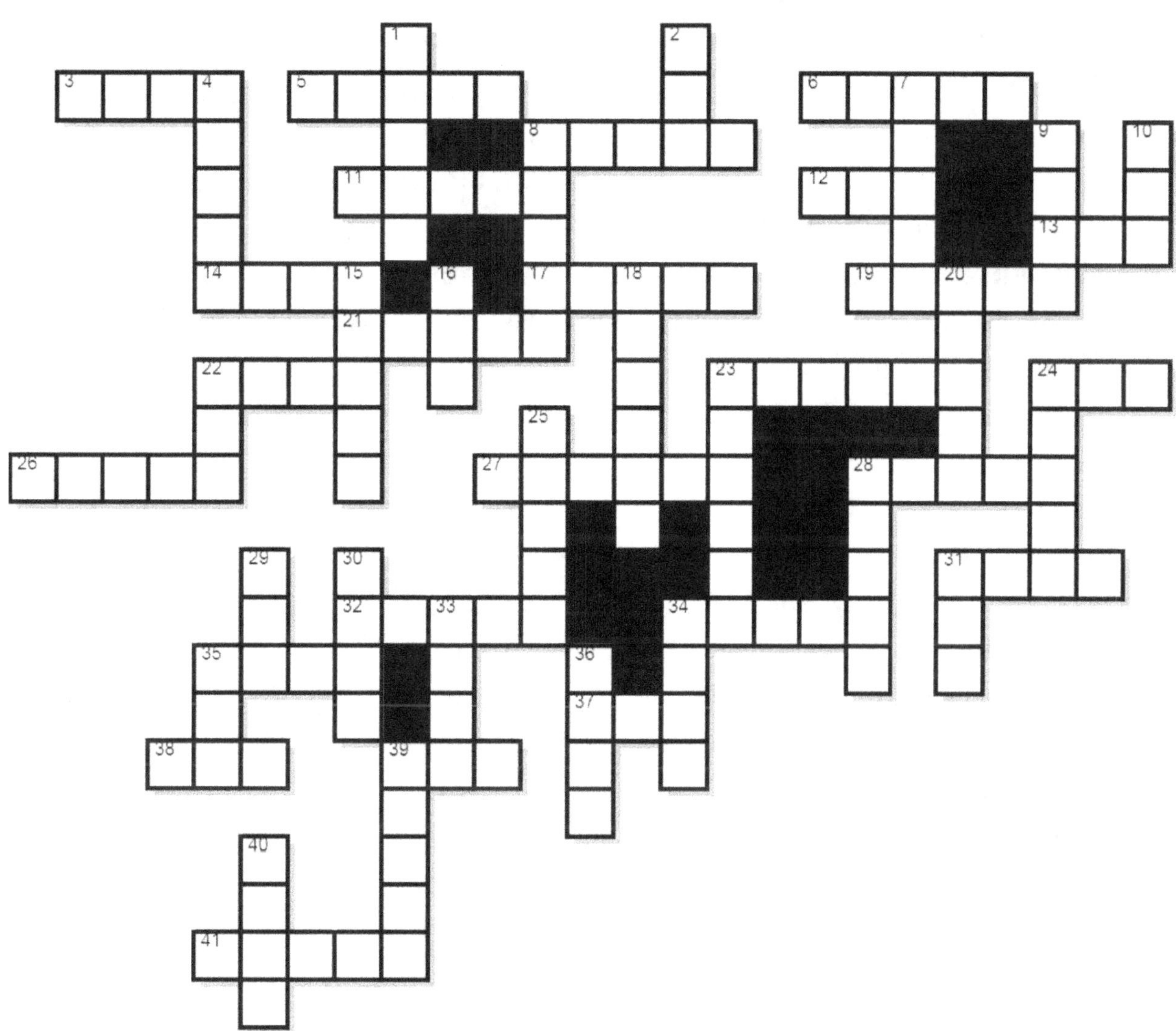

Across

3. Don't drink. ____ your juice!
5. Best hydration tool
6. Many vitamins put together in one of these ____ vitamins
8. This pea makes Hummus
11. Latin dance or a dip
12. Apple cider vinnegar (abbrev.)
13. An ocean weed?
14. Cold pressed olives (abbrev.)
17. Eat one every day
19. Short for fermented cabbage
21. Prefix pertaining to the brain
22. An Asian longevity berry
23. A type of fresh water
24. HydroxyTryptoPhan (abbrev.)
26. What do frugivores eat?
27. Ask your ______.
28. Ezekiel is a sprouted kind.
31. Carrots and beets are a type.
32. Important body fluid (not blood)
34. There are nine essential ______ acids.
35 Gamma AminoButyric Acid (abbrev.)
37. Prefix for the new type of genetic study.
38. Shorthand for Magnesium
39. A leafy green: ___ choy
41. A yellow fruit you can use to alkalize your water.

Down

1. Cook using this water method
2. N-Acetyl Cysteine (abbrev.)
4. Avoid many foods this color
7. Internal body detox center
8. Chocolate comes from beans
9. Get plenty of nighttime ____
10. Have a cup in the afternoon.
15. Good source of sulfur that smells good when grilled.
16. Get this kind of ___ shine!
18. These items are the basis of the SPOM! Diet
20. Great protein, otherwise known as pond scum.
22. This lower part of your body serves as another brain.
23. Shorthand for 'mushy' fungus
24. Prefix for water
25. Slang for Kombucha
28. Try a diet free from this animal fluid.
29. Essential Fatty Acids (abbrev.)
30. Seed source of Omega3s
31. Uncooked foods are ___.
33. Fermented soy paste
34. Balances alkaline
35. Gamma Linolenic Acid (abbrev.)
36. Sweet Potatoes have ____ carotene.
39. Popular color for good rice
40. Advanced Glycation Endproducts (abbrev.)

NUTRITION PLAN

Sometimes when we get busy, it is easy to forget to make healthy choices. If you have a chart of healthy options and ideas available, then when you're hungry and your brain may not be working efficiently to make highest and best choices, you have a list to fall back on. Look over the pages in the SPOM Text where you circled foods that appealed to you. Write these foods and menu ideas for your meals throughout the day. Then make sure you keep these foods and snacks in your pantry!

Meal Time	Food and Snack Ideas
Breaking the fast	
Morning Snacks	
Midday Meal	
Afternoon Snacks	
Evening Meal	
Evening Snacks	
Bedtime Treats	

OH POOP!

Everybody poops! How often do you take on this fun task? Ideally, you should be evacuating your bowels shortly after every single time you have a meal. Yes. Really. So start to notice just how many times a day do you go. If you are not "fasting mode" and it is not at least once or more a day, this might clue you in to a toxic plugged-up bowel. Failure to eliminate waster might result in 'waste' or toxins leaking out in other places – like your skin! See how many times you poop for at least a couple of days. What's the consistency of it? Is it easy going and mildly firm? Loose and watery? So hard, you think you might blow a circuit?

Get over being uncomfortable about this. Seriously, this is truly important for you to start noticing. Your life could depend on it.

Day and Time	Consistency	Other Notes

BTW, there are lots of things you can do to help get things moving down there, like exercise and water, especially eating better, including more raw foods and fiber in your diet, plus hydrating properly, and most of all *moving* your body!

MAKE-UP CYPHER

See how many personal care products you can identify in this cypher. If the products share the same letters, then they will be the same across all the words. These are names of very common products. See how many you can guess?

Use the alphabet at the bottom to keep track of your code and get decoding James or Jane Bond! *HINT: Letter "F" in the box gets decoded to an "A."*

Answers on Page 130

| D | X | FA | R |

| K | X | Q | X | V | E | Z |

| A | Z | X | A | Z | U | FA | E | M |

| D | B | FA | N | R | X | X |

| Q | S | R | L | FA | Q | N |

| K | X | E | A | S | M | S | X | E | Z | U |

| N | X | S | D | M | G | U | S | C | Z | U |

| M | X | X | M | B | R | FA | D | M | Z |

| X | S | Q |

| O | X | G | E | A | FA | M | S | X | E |

A=__ B=__ C=__ D=__ E=__ F=A G=__ H=__ I=__ K=__ L=__ M=__

N=__ O=__ P=__ Q=__ R=__ S=__ T=__ U=__ V=__ X=__ Z=__

PRODUCT INVENTORY

Please go into your bathroom, kitchen, bedroom, purse and/or car and write down a list of every single personal care product you own. This means makeup-shampoo, deodorant, moisturizer, perfumes, everything. You may have to write pretty small to fit everything in here. I also have a feeling you will need multiple sheets of paper to do this one, so get some extra paper! (Or make copies of the following page.)

This is a good time to do a nice major cleaning of your bath shelves. And see if perhaps you have developed a shopping addiction to compensate for your self-harming problems?

Write down product names and manufacturers, along with the purpose of the product. Most importantly, note how often you actually use the product (daily-weekly-monthly-rarely). Then finally look at the list of ingredients and count the total number of ingredients in each product.

Make special note if you understand what each and every ingredient is and what it does. (Yes or no answer.) Then finally, make a comment on whether you would be willing to remove, or at least replace that product with a different healthier version. (Yes, no or maybe answer.)

Product +Maker	Purpose	Times Used?	Number of Ingredients	Understand Ingredients?	Replace? Release?
Example: Argan Oil by BioExtra	*Face moisture*	*Daily*	*1*	*Yes!*	*No way!*

Product +Maker	Purpose	Times Used?	Number of Ingredients	Understand Ingredients?	Replace? Release?

Ingredient Inventory

Make a list of every single ingredient you came across that you did not recognize or understand what it was or what it did. Either look at the ingredients mentioned in the main SPOM! text or go online and do some research and see what you can find out. Make sure the ingredient is actually needed in your products (other than to make is cheaper or make it go further). Make sure it is healthy for you, has no adverse side effects, or worse may be contributing to your breakouts!

Ingredient	What it does and possible side effects

Meditation – A Mindful Meal

How do you feel about your favorite foods? Whether or not they are healthy for you, do you have an intimate emotional relationship with any particular culinary delight? Cheese? French Fries? Chocolate? Wine? Sour Dough Bread? Pasta? A good cup of Coffee? Most humans are food addicts and we don't even know it. We eat for more than hunger and for energy. We eat emotionally.

As explained in the main SPOM text, we acquire other emotionally-charged brain chemicals from foods. On top of that, when you are tense or anxious, your digestive system can get really riled up. It can put your whole system into survival mode, in essence shutting proper digestion down. So what are you to do?

You can start to do all the typical things. Learn about nutrition. Read labels. Don't buy things if you don't understand the ingredients. Shop in stores and eat at restaurants you trust to supply more healthy options.

You can also begin to be extra meditatively mindful of your meals. This meditation does not require you to be in a quiet dark room. You do it wherever and whenever you find yourself about to eat. The parameters are this: no chit-chat, TV, radio, cellphone, reading material or other media external stimulus allowed. Try to sit alone when you eat, or eat with a partner who also wishes to be mindful of their meal. Other than that, the meditation is just about you and your food: like you might concentrate on the breath in a typical meditation - here you concentrate on the consumption process.

Begin

Begin by blessing the food in front of you. Be thankful of every stage that food had to come through to get in front of you. The seed company, the soil amendment company, the farmer, the harvesters, processors, packing and distribution companies, the truckers, the merchants, the traders, the market personnel, the buyers, the cook, and the servers, not to mention some miraculous power that allows food to grow in the first place. Thank it all.

Before you take your first bite, really look at the food on your plate. Enjoy the different shapes, sizes and colors. Enjoy the aroma that may be wafting up. When you finally take a small first bite, hear the sound of the utensil on the plate or bowl. Then hear how the food sounds inside your mouth cavity as you chew. Feel how it feels against your teeth and the roof of your mouth. Is it hot or cold or just right? Really enjoy the sensation of the flavor in your mouth. Chew it until your food is completely liquefied. As you continue to take more bites, continue this same sensational ritual awareness throughout the whole process.

Notice how the food feels going down your esophagus. And see if you can be in touch with your stomach and notice when it starts to feel full. Lay your hand on your stomach and say a thankful thought to your body for taking such good care of you. Take a pause between each set of bites and take a calm deep breath and see how relaxed you can get.

When your meal is finally over, feel the feeling of being satiated in a way you've never noticed before. Do you feel more relaxed? More at ease? Notice any additional cravings you right have after the meal? Do you desire sugar or caffeine? Before you attend to that craving, take another pause. Look around at your surroundings and try to take in all of the details around you. When you were hungry and about to eat, they were probably not as much in focus. Do they seem more in focus now? Notice how you feel emotionally when you are done eating.

If you decide to give in to after-meal cravings, make sure you take the same mindful enjoyment-focused approach to that part of your meal as well.

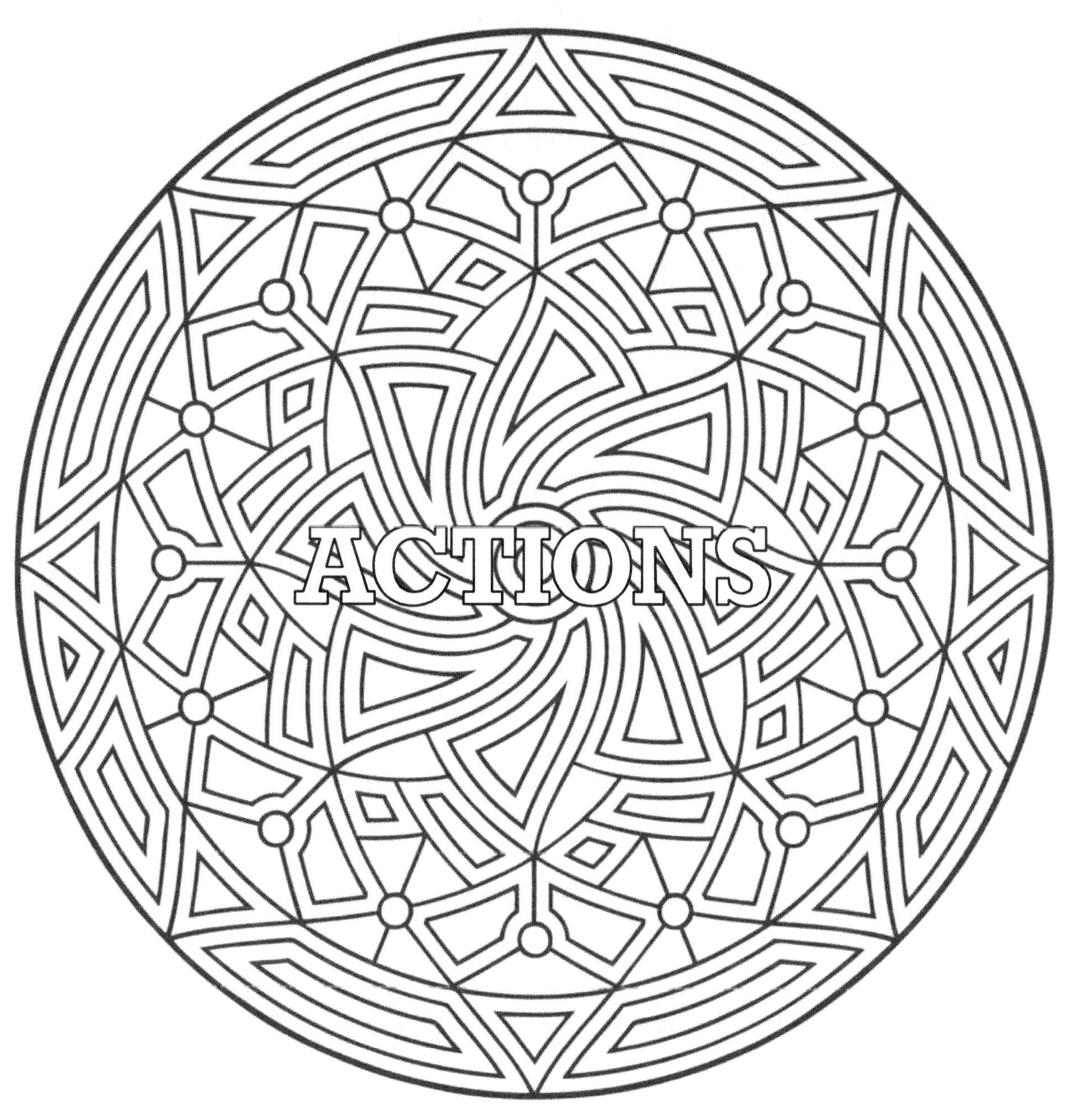

Color Me Powerful.

REWARD WORKSHEETS

Here are some nice things that you can do for yourself to reward non-picking behavior. Circle the ones that sound good to you.

- Get an acupuncture or acupressure treatment
- Doodle, draw or paint
- Play your favorite music
- Scrapbook
- Go for a walk or a jog
- Play with a favorite healing bedroom toy
- Get some chiropractic care
- Do some energy healing, including self-Reiki
- Do a flotation tank
- Knit or crochet
- Have a heartfelt conversation with a friend
- Sing in the shower
- Get into the sunlight for some light therapy
- Play a game.
- Buy yourself something special that you have saved up for
- Have massage or bodywork done
- Dance
- Do some deep breathing and rebirth yourself
- Write a poem
- Listen to sound healing sounds like Tibetan or crystal singing bowls
- Tap tap tap on your healing meridians
- Look at (or kiss) your beloved
- Whistle a happy tune

CREATE YOUR OWN REWARDS

Add you own comments and little notes around this diagram of things of the rewards you like from the previous page, or add other things that you can do that will support these three areas in your life:

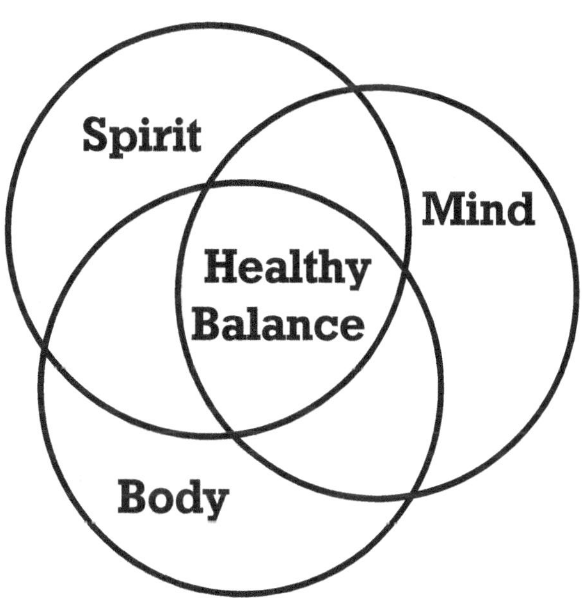

COMPETING HABIT LIST

Going back to your Breakout Journal and Habit Assessment Chart and also use some of the items from your Reward Worksheet, make a chart of potential scenarios where you might self-harm and notate a specific action plan that you will commit to trying before you go to pick.

You're going to lick the habit… i.e. lick the pick (groan)!

- Can you name the emotion you are feeling immediately before you reach up for your face or other self-harming spot?

- If you cannot name that emotion, look at the Feeling Faces towards the beginning of this workbook, or use some other method to get in touch with what is going on.
  This is critical. You gotta STOP-LOOK-LISTEN to what is happening in your heart.

- What else can you do to make yourself feel better and express where you are at emotionally?

- How else can you release the internal tension you are grappling with?

- What can you do to get back in touch with a bigger better reality than the one that pushes you towards self-harm?

- What other thing can you do to get a rush of adrenaline or opiates?

- How else can you communicate what's going on inside of you?

This is one list that you want to commit to memory and keep it (or your Reward Worksheet) handy on your desk, fridge or phone, so when your brain freezes up and wants to go into the old "Feel-Good" Loop pattern, you have a cheat sheet to get you outta there fast.

Habit Competition

Typical time/location of habit	What I will do first or instead
Example: After I brush my teeth at night I lean into the mirror to do close inspection of skin.	*Example: I'll brush my teeth over the kitchen sink. Then I will stretch and touch my toes five times.*

HABIT CHANGE MAZE

Take a break from the hard thinking work and have fun with this puzzle!
See if you can avoid the negative effects of self-harm? I bet you can!
Start at "NOW" and get to Recovery!
Like life, there is *more than one* winning path through this maze!

Answer on Page 131

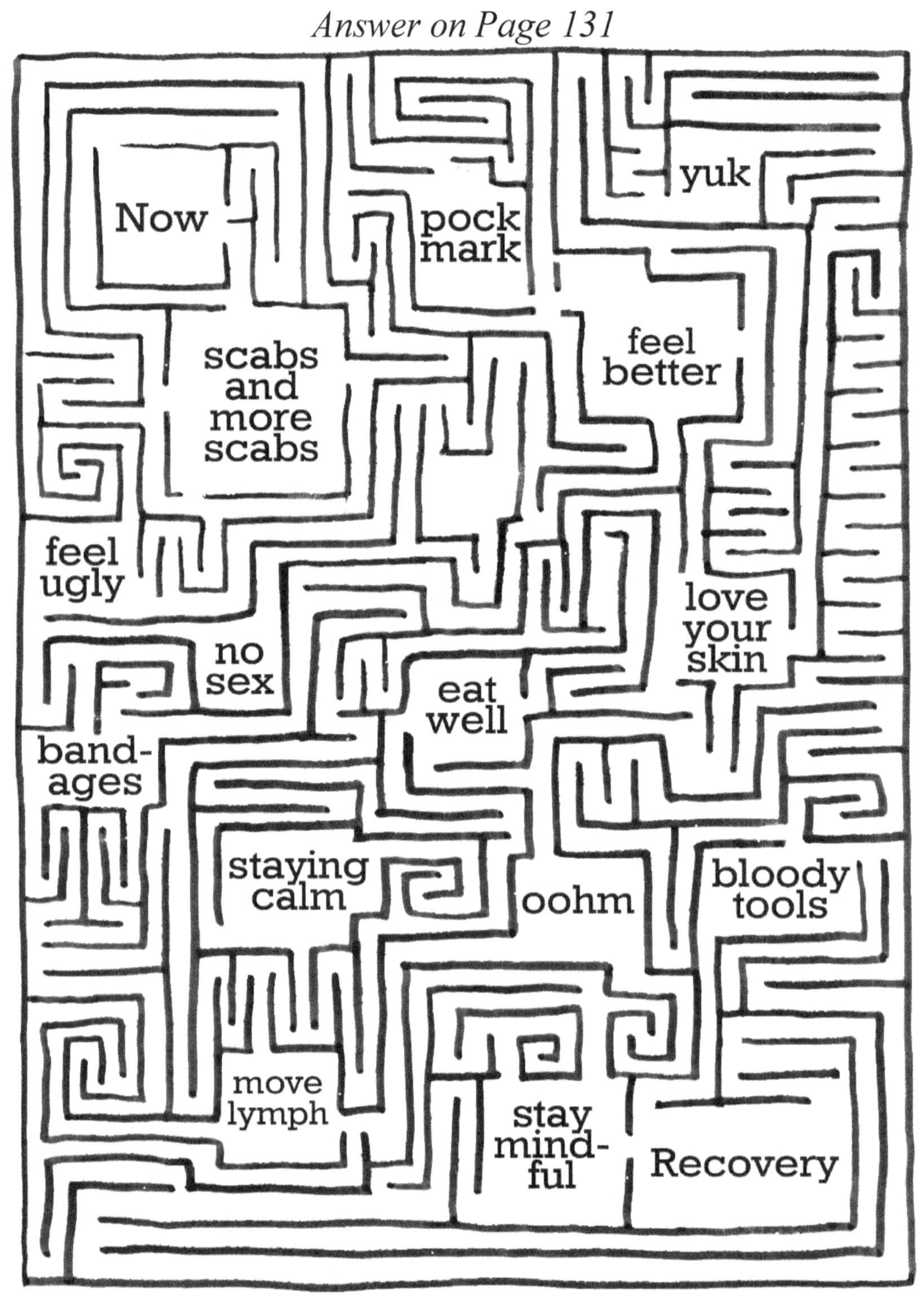

DAILY SCHEDULE

Maintain a regular daily schedule to add *structure* to your life. Include the very basic daily stuff: taking vitamins, brushing your teeth, saying good night prayers, etc. When you are feeling anxious, you will KNOW what to do next based on your schedule. The schedule will help you remember to DO the basics, and if you can at cross off some of basics things, you will feel a sense of accomplishment at the end of your day.

Time	Basic Things to Do
Wake Up	Say Affirmations and Review Gratitude List Take Three Deep Breaths and Make Your Bed
Morning	Break Your Fast Slowly Get Groomed: shave, brush and floss Exercise, Stretch, Walk, Movement
Later Morning	Light "Breaking the Fast" Food
Noon	Say Grace Vitamins and Minerals with Food
Afternoon	Tea or Yerba Mate, Light Snacks
Sundown	Get Grounded and Stretch
Dinner	Say Grace Vitamins and Minerals with Food
Bedtime	Non-Caffeinated Tea Moisturize, Brush and Floss Say Affirmations and Review Gratitude List

WEEKLY SCHEDULE

Create a weekly schedule with things that support your recovery. If you think you don't have enough time to do yoga? How about you commit to yoga one day a week and make that day, say… Monday? How about a weekly cleaning or home organization night? Are you getting out in nature on a regular basis? Schedule time! Include a day of rest, whether it's Sunday or another day. You deserve time off for good behavior. Stick to your schedule so that it becomes a priority, and then a habit.

Day	Things to Do
Monday	
Tuesday	
Wednesday	
Thursday	
Friday	
Saturday	
Sunday	

<u>Attitude Adjustment Chart</u>

Think beyond 'picking.' What other stress responses do you exhibit? How do you react when someone cuts you off on the road? When you drop something accidentally? When someone does something questionable at work? When a loved one looks at you sideways? Write down your typical angry or resentful response and then see if you can find a silver lining to the event and write how you would respond if you saw it differently.

Stressful Event	My Typical Response	Conscious Response
Example: *Someone cut me off on the freeway.*	*Example:* *Flip them off and curse them.*	*Example:* *Say a grateful prayer for your fast reflexes.*

SWOT Analysis

In the corporate world, they often use a process called a "SWOT" analysis to define "Strengths-Weakness-Opportunities-Threats." We have already discussed your Weakness and Threats in quite a bit of detail. Now let's turn the tables.

Life is on your side.

You are still alive and somehow were led to find this book so that you could explore healing. Now that you have some plans in mind, let's look a little more closely at your "Strengths" and then we'll look at your "Opportunities."

Take a moment to list a few of your short and long range goals:

Intellectual Goals

____

____

Physical Goals

____

____

Spiritual Goals

____

____

Emotional Goals

____

____

My Strengths & Assets

You can have great circumstances and a lousy attitude no matter what is going on. Or you can have lousy circumstances and a great attitude to what is going on around you. Focus on the good. Take a moment to write some positive asset about each of these elements in your life.

My Mind

____

____

My Body

____

____

My Spirit

____

____

My Emotions

____

____

My Friends
(and Acquaintances that could become friends in the future)

____

____

My Neighbor and Neighborhood

____

____

My Community and Places where I belong

____

____

My City

____

My State

____

My Nation

____

My World

____

My Universe

____

My Opportunities

Look at these same areas of your life. Where are the opportunities for you to expand? Where and how can you contribute to greater potential in each of these areas?

My Mind

____

____

My Body

____

____

My Spirit

____

____

My Emotions

____

____

My Friends
(and Acquaintances that could become friends in the future)

____

____

____

My Neighbor and Neighborhood

____

____

My Community and Places where I belong

____

____

____

My City

____

My State

____

My Nation

____

My World

____

My Universe

____

MEDITATION – ANCHORING

In Neuro Linguistic Programming (NLP) therapy, a coach might work with you to help you remember a time in your life when you felt happy and powerful. It is important to have these memories, because they give your strength, hope and courage to move forward productively in life. If you don't have an NLP coach handy at the moment, you can try this technique out on yourself.

Frankly, as a self-harmer, you might be feeling despondent and like you have never been happy and powerful in your life. But trust me, if those memories don't come right away (they may be buried) they're there. Have you ever seen a toddler take their first steps in life on their own two feet? There is a look of joy, shock, independence and incredulous wonder on their face while they get the hang of it. At the very least, we know that happened to you once. And now that you are open to the idea, you will uncover more of these moments in your life.

Get into a quiet space and a meditative state of mind. Let your higher consciousness know that you're open to remembering moments when you felt really positive about your life. Allow yourself time to recollect. Nothing needs to be forced. Once you get an impression. Try to witness all of the sensory feelings around that memory (sight, sound, taste, touch, smells, feelings) and embrace the moment as fully as you can. Now find a very specific spot on your body (hand, arm, head, anywhere). It should be someplace that you have easy access to at any given moment. Use your dominant hand to do this. I.e., if you are right handed, use your right hand to touch, and if left-handed, use your left. Feel the intense positive feelings around that memory and tap or touch in that spot. When you do that, let the ecstasy of positivity flood your being. You are anchoring your memory.

Now anytime you feel out of control or depressed, touch that spot and access those feelings and remind yourself that whatever you are currently going through is only a bump on the road. It is *not* the definition of your life or who you are.

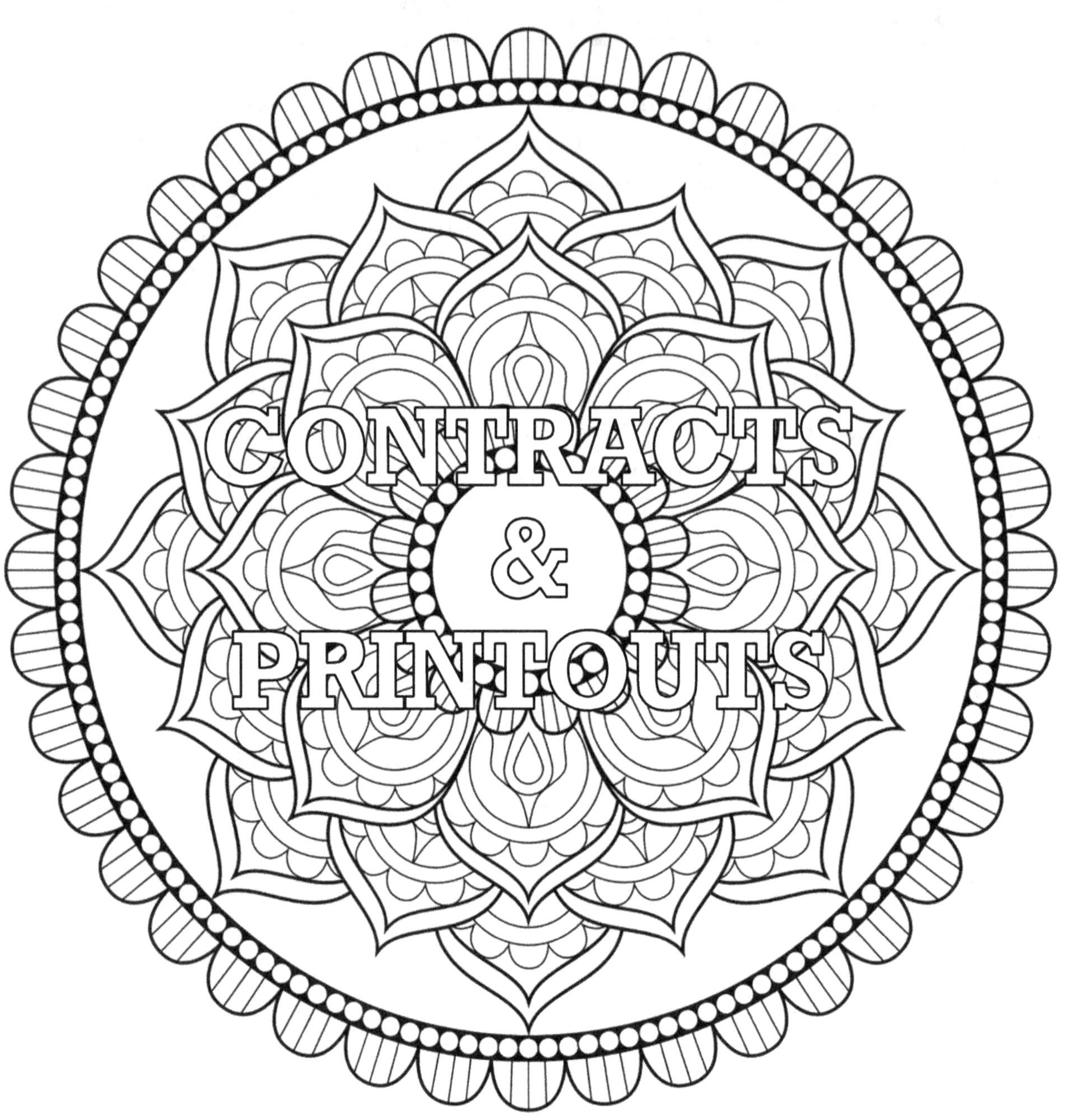

Color Me Appreciated.

My Support Team

Make sure you have a 'phone list' of people you can reach out to around the clock and find support when you run into tough situations. Remember that not everyone is an early riser or a night owl. Know which person is the best person to contact at different times of day or night. And also remember to reach out when you have good times, too. Share your wins and happiness.

Team   **Best Way to Contact**   **Best Time**

AGREEMENTS

Copy and paste the following agreements so that you can have a clean blank master copy in the book and then make changes or additions as your condition or scenario changes.

First of all, you should have something in writing with yourself that lets yourself know you mean business. So copy the self-agreement, sign and date it and put it with your other important papers and contracts.

Next, as you build your support team, make a pact with them that they will support your positive future and have them sign and date the Support Team Agreement. Talk over all the point of the agreement so you are both in consensus on all of the points.

Likewise, agreements go two ways. So you as the person in recovery will need to offer some agreements back to your support team. Sign and date those as well and give them a copy.

Contractual Breaches and Disputes

So what happens if one or both of you do not hold up your ends of the agreement(s). This should be discussed when you first enter into the agreements. Agree ahead of time on some consequences and remedies for contract infringements. Some therapies actually suggest negative reinforcement or humiliating ramifications. I suggest doing something positive. I prefer a carrot over a stick.

- Money Restitution: You could have a jar where quarters or dollars go whenever there is a breach. Make sure that this money ends up going to a charitable cause, so neither party benefits financially from slips.

- Reformation: This is when you both agree there were fundamental issues with the contract and you agree to re-write some of the terms.

- Specific Performance Orders: Perhaps you will have to perform an unpleasant chore for the aggrieved party, extra babysitting, shoveling snow, making dinner, or you name it.

SELF-AGREEMENT

I, _________________________________, hereby agree to the following:

- I will accept myself for the unique individual that I am now and I am becoming.

- I will learn to recognize the symptoms of slips and not beat myself up for set-backs.

- I will not take other people's decisions or actions personally.

- I will use whatever tools within my capability and at my disposal to keep myself on a healing path. That means saying affirmations, doing reading and writing, and sticking to whatever reasonable plans and goals I have set up for myself.

- I will allow myself to reevaluate those plans and goals to make sure they are still reasonable and do not put undue stress or excessive pressure on me.

- I will allow myself to de-compress and de-stress, and have a complete do nothing, goof-off day once a week every week. This is non-negotiable. I need a break.

- I will be vigilant in choosing healthier food choices and I will pursue my highest and best health choices for the remainder of my life.

- I will accept graciously support from wherever it comes from and not question the motives of people helping me out.

- I will be crystal clear in my communications and speak with integrity to everyone I meet.

Signed,

_________________________________   _________________________________
                                          Date

____
Print Name

SUPPORT TEAM AGREEMENT

Support Team Member Copy

I, _________________________________, hereby agree to the following:

- I will be a Support Team Member for the following individual:

  ____.

- I will accept you for the unique individual that you are and are becoming.

- I will not put unnecessary demands on your time or energy.

- I will learn to recognize that the symptoms of slips and never beat you up for set-backs. And I will not take your decisions or actions personally.

- Rather, when you feel discouraged, I will remind you of the positive traits that you possess (that you may have forgotten) and remind you of the goals you have and those you have achieved.

- I will support your choices to eat healthier and not try to tempt you with items that we both know are not for your highest and best good.

- I will be more considerate of your feelings.

- If I have doubts, I will keep them to myself, as they are only mine and not yours.

Signed,

_________________________________   _________________________________
                                          Date

____
Print Name

SUPPORT TEAM AGREEMENT

Person in Recovery Copy

I, _________________________________, hereby agree to the following:

- I will graciously accept the support from the following individual:

  _________________________________.

  I will accept your support and not question your motives for helping me out.

- I will not put unnecessary demands on your time or energy unless I am really in dire need of support.

- I will not take your decisions or actions personally.

- I will not impose my choices to eat healthier on you in exchange for your unconditional support for my choices.

- I will be more considerate of how *you* must feel being around someone who has hurt themselves.

- I will be crystal clear in my communications and I will not play games and withhold my feelings when you ask about them.

Signed,

____

____
Date

____
Print Name

AFFIRMATIONS

The following next few pages are for you to copy or tear out of the book (carefully) and putting them up someplace prominent in your world. Hit the thrift store or dollar store and grab a couple of affordable 8.5 x 11 frames (these are usually called document frames). If you have a tough time finding those, you can always cut these printouts down to 8x10 size and sometimes those frames are easier to find

As far as the affirmations go, you can frame them just in black and white as they are, or I am casually suggesting that you color, doodle and draw around the words and make them your own, or cut out some pleasing pictures from magazines and paste them around the words.

I AM IN MY BODY:
FRONT TO BACK,
SIDE TO SIDE,
HEAD TO TOE,
FACING FORWARD,
WITH BOTH FEET
ON THE GROUND,
STARING STRAIGHT AHEAD.

*I take full responsibility
for all the areas of my life I have created
and respect the unique path I have taken
to where I am now.*

*I know inherently that everything works
out for my Highest Good.*

*I take every opportunity available
to Up-Level my life in terms of how I respond
to everyday stress, what I eat, how I act,
what I think, and how I feel.*

*I am grateful to have upgraded insight
on how to improve my health and my life.*

*I breathe and relax in this now moment,
knowing that my natural evolution
is unfolding in a perfectly fascinating
and wonderful manner.*

I INTEND TO BE
OF WHOLE AND SANE MIND.

I INTEND TO BE
WHOLE AND VIBRANT IN BODY.

I INTEND TO SING MY SONG
AND LIVE MY LIFE
FOR ALL IT'S WORTH!

CERTIFICATIONS

In typical twelve step programs, they focus on people admitting they go back to the first step if they have a slip. You have to get a "newcomer" chip" all over again. Not in my program, baby. Of course, you may have to go back to re-committing and practicing fundamental stuff in your program, but that does not negate the positive strides you have taken.

As far as your commencement papers. I want you to take these seriously. Once you have made it through an entire hour without obsessing and self-harm, get that first certificate in a frame and up on a wall or on your desk or bedside. Look at in regularly knowing that you made it for that amount of time. It's a big deal. You deserve to be proud of that.

Once you have made it past the hour and made it successfully through an entire half-day, twelve hour period, turn the paper over and make the half day certification the visible certificate. No matter what happens after that day forward, this is the level you are at. I do not care if you have a slip and go back to picking every hour on the hour! I want you to acknowledge that you DID make it through that half day. That is how this world works.

Hey, I graduated from UCLA. Now if I decided to go back to community college and take some remedial courses, does that take away from my degree? Should I take my diploma down? No. Of course not. So likewise, once you have reached a goal. It is yours forever. Remind yourself of that win by framing it.

Keep track of your progress and upgrade the certificate that you display as you move forward.

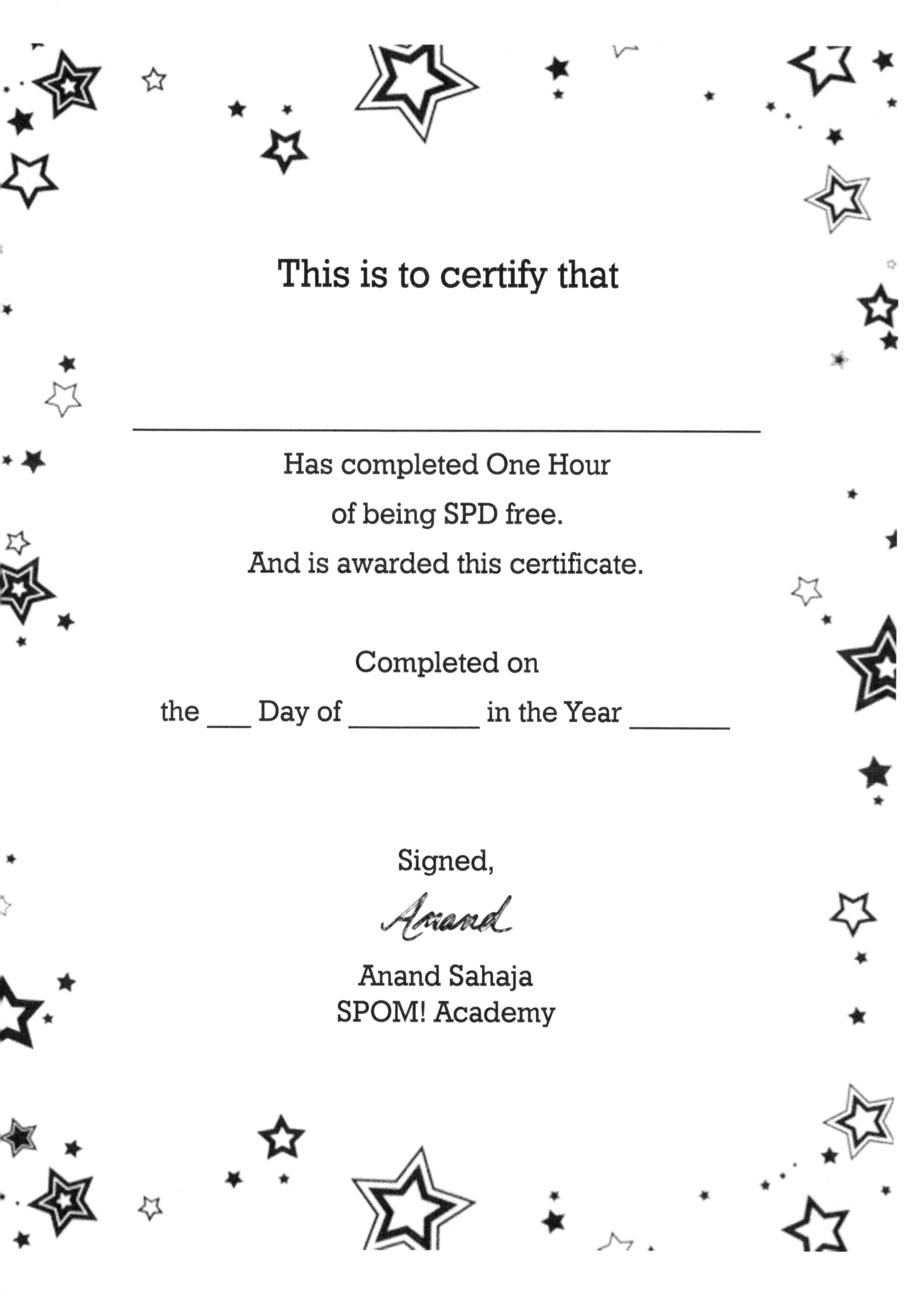

This is to certify that

____

Has completed One Hour
of being SPD free.
And is awarded this certificate.

Completed on
the ___ Day of _________ in the Year _______

Signed,

Anand Sahaja
SPOM! Academy

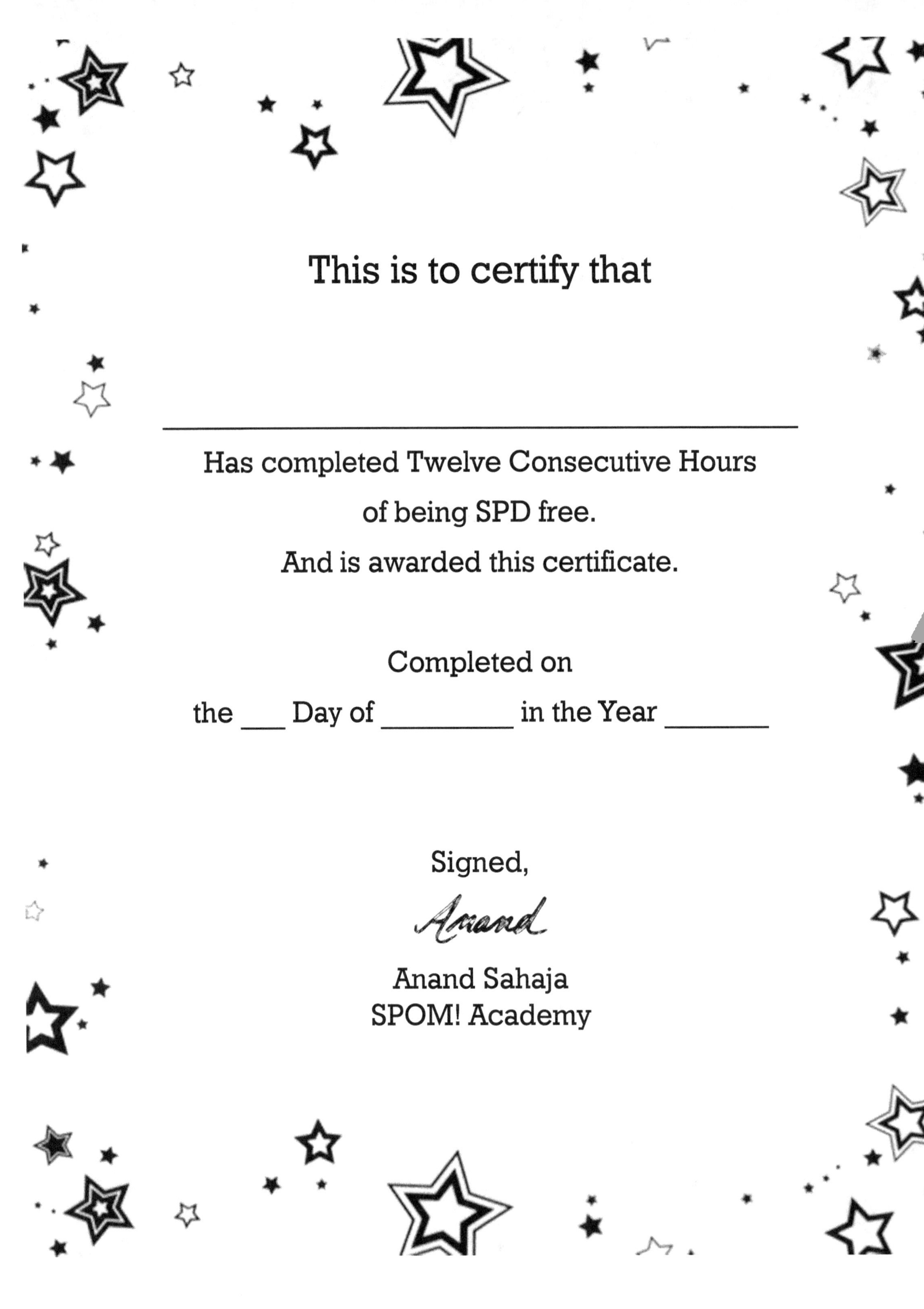

This is to certify that

____

Has completed Twelve Consecutive Hours
of being SPD free.
And is awarded this certificate.

Completed on
the ___ Day of _________ in the Year _______

Signed,

Anand Sahaja
SPOM! Academy

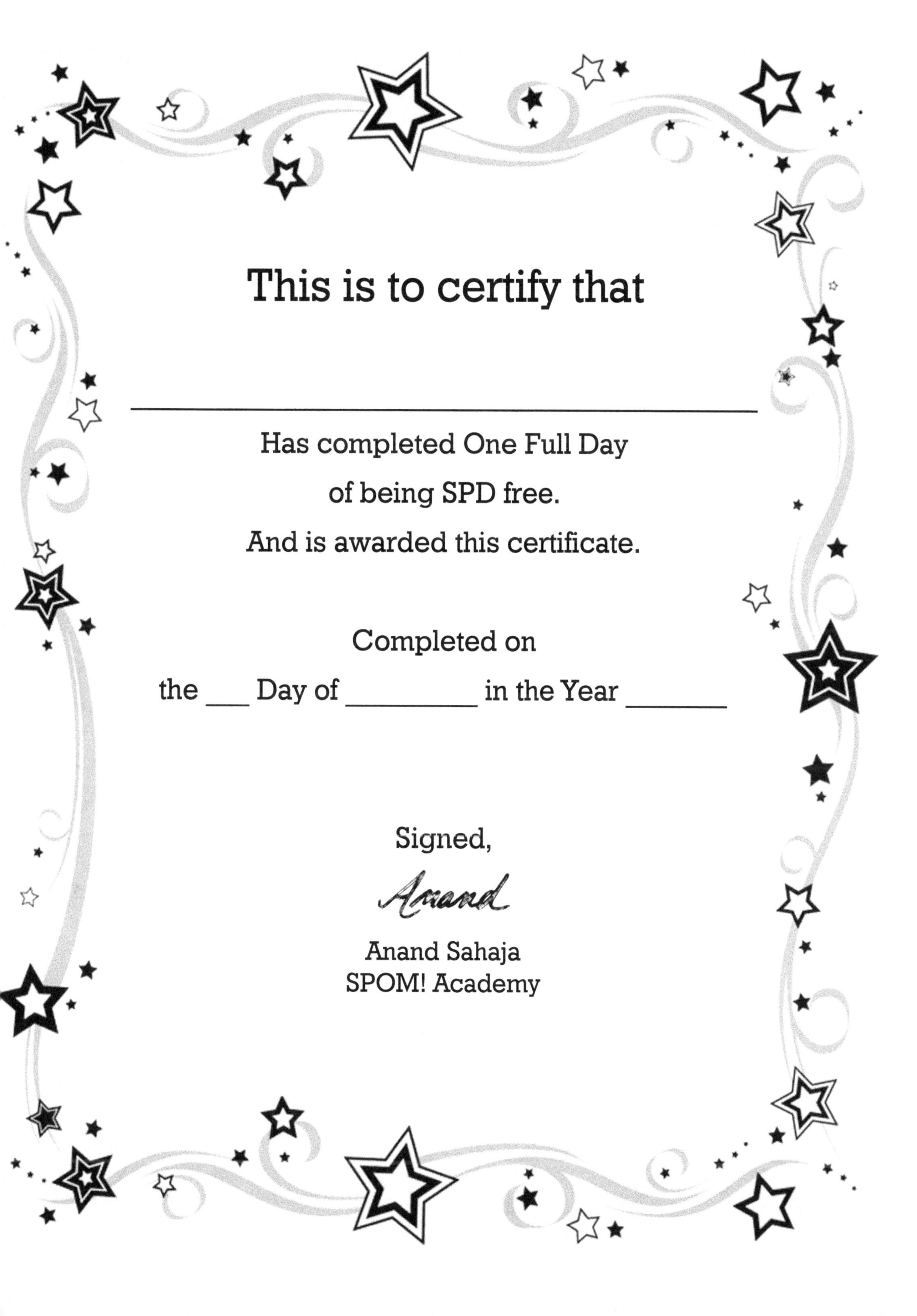

This is to certify that

____

Has completed One Full Day

of being SPD free.

And is awarded this certificate.

Completed on

the ___ Day of _________ in the Year _______

Signed,

Anand Sahaja
SPOM! Academy

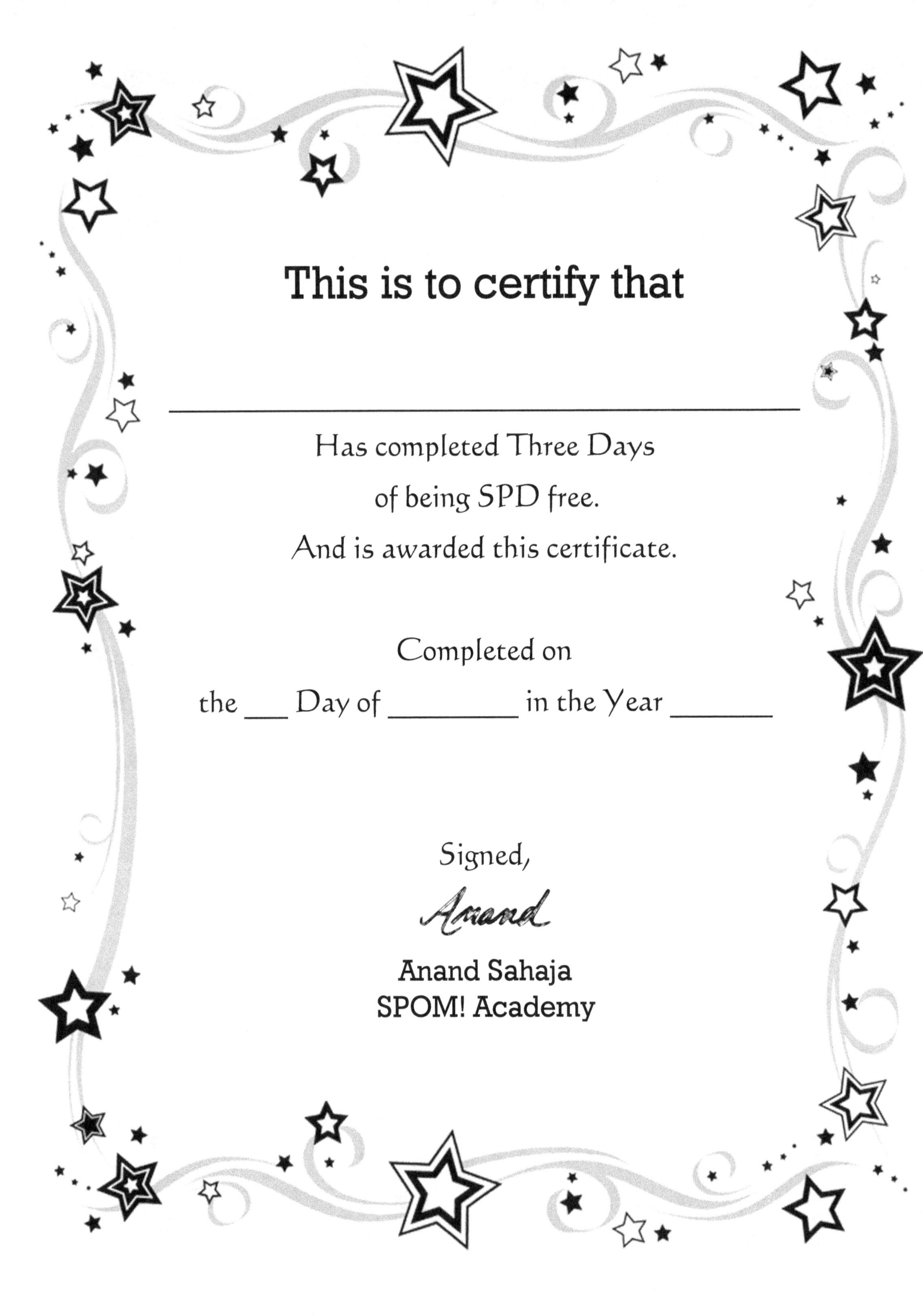

This is to certify that

____

Has completed Three Days
of being SPD free.
And is awarded this certificate.

Completed on

the ___ Day of _________ in the Year _______

Signed,

Anand

Anand Sahaja
SPOM! Academy

This Certifies that

____

Has completed One Full Week of being SPD free.
And is awarded this certificate.

Completed on

the ___ Day of _________ in the Year _______

Signed,

Anand

Anand Sahaja
SPOM! Academy

This Certifies that

____

Has completed Two Weeks of being SPD free.

And is awarded this certificate.

Completed on

the ___ Day of __________ in the Year ________

Signed,

Anand

Anand Sahaja
SPOM! Academy

This is to Certify that

____

Has completed Three Weeks of being SPD free.

And is awarded this certificate

.

Completed on

the ___ Day of _________ in the Year _______

Signed,

Anand

Anand Sahaja
SPOM! Academy

This is to Certify that

____

Has completed A COMPLETE MONTH of being SPD free.

And is awarded this certificate.

Completed on

the ___ Day of _________ in the Year _______

Signed,

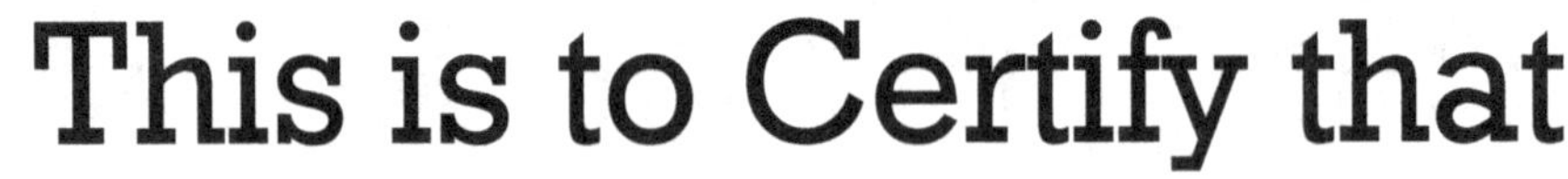

Anand Sahaja
SPOM! Academy

This Certifies

____

Has completed Three Months of being SPD free.
And is awarded this certificate.

Completed on
the ___ Day of _________ in the Year _______

Signed,

Anand

Anand Sahaja
SPOM! Academy

This Certifies

____

Has completed Six Months of being SPD free.

And is awarded this certificate.

Completed on

the ___ Day of _________ in the Year _______

Signed,

Anand

**Anand Sahaja
SPOM! Academy**

This Certifies that

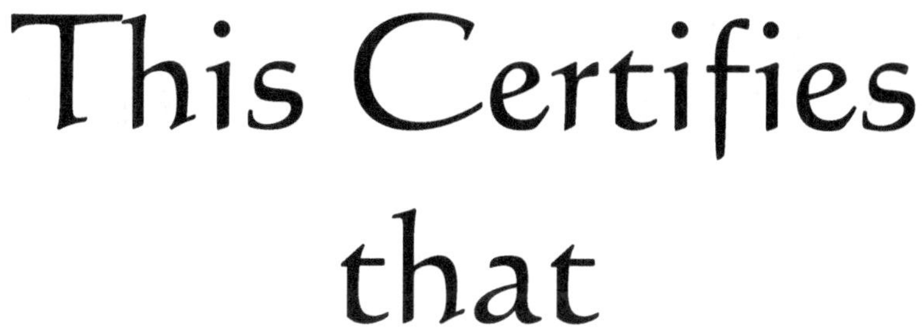

____

Has given birth to a new person and
completed Nine Months of being SPD free.

And is awarded this certificate.

Completed on

the ___ Day of _________ in the Year _______

Signed,

**Anand Sahaja
SPOM! Academy**

This Certifies
that

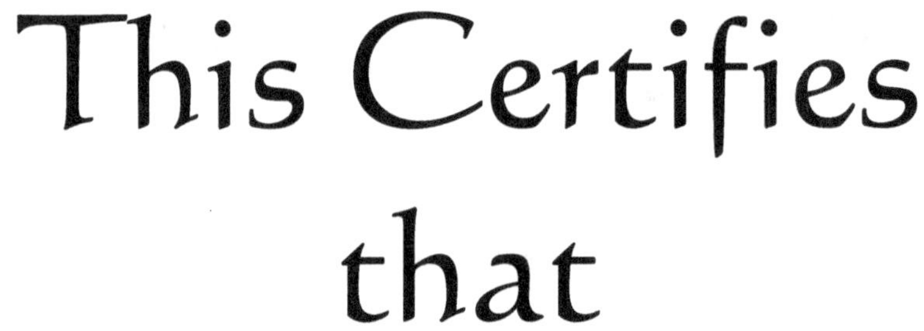

____

Has completed One full Year
of being SPD free.

And is awarded this certificate.

Completed on

the ___ Day of _________ in the Year _______

Signed,

Anand

**Anand Sahaja
SPOM! Academy**

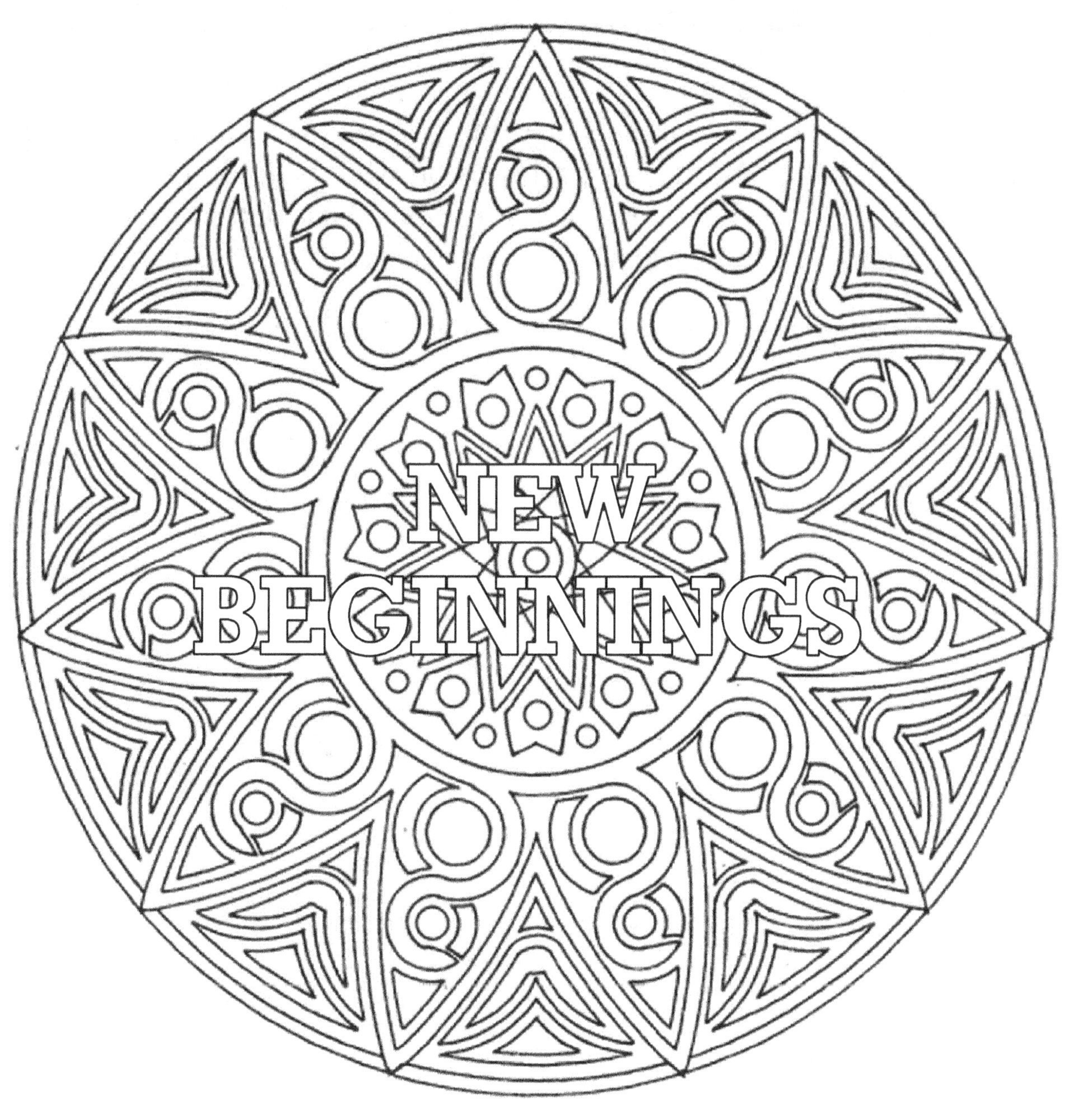

Color Me Healing.

What's Holding You Up?

Normally you hear a similar phrase, "What's holding you back?" We've looked at a good deal of those things. I want you to focus on the foundations of your future success. Focus on what is holding you up! Label the table legs with your assets or reasons that you know you have that will enable you to be successful in recovery.

(You can also add more extensions and legs to the table!)

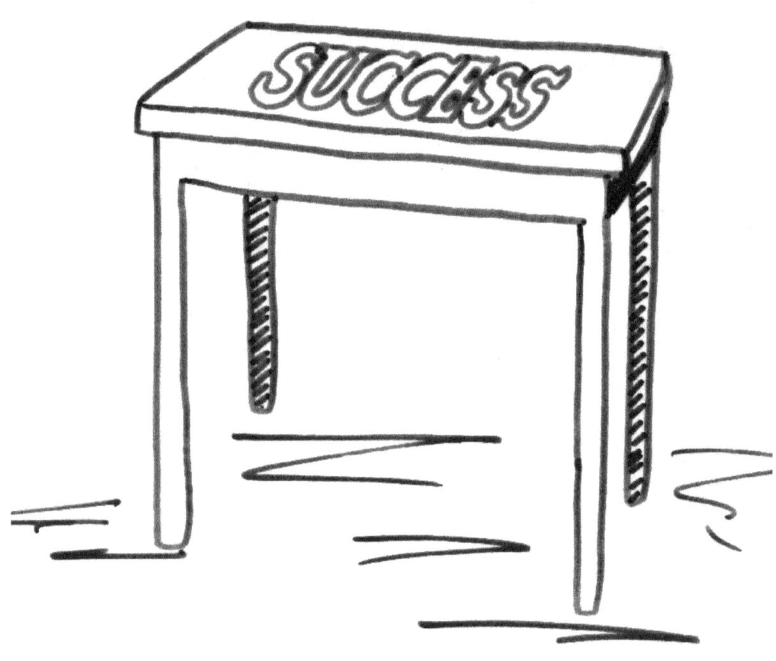

WORD BENEFITS GAME

Answer all of the clues below. Then transfer the letters from the clues into the appropriate boxes in the grid below. Fill out the remaining clues below to fill in the remaining spaces above and get a nice affirmation to remember on a daily basis. I have started the puzzle out by providing you with all of the letters "A" and a couple of other letters.

Answers on Page 131

	A	B	C	D	E	F	G	H	I	J	K	L	M	N	O	P
1				A						A						
2	A															A
3									A					A		

(If there is an xx underneath a line in a clue,
it simply means that letter is not in the final top affirmation.)

The state of being you will be in when no longer chained by bad habits. (Also a Pharrell Williams song!)

___ ___ ___ ___ ___ ___ ___
B3 C3 P3 I2 I1 F1 H3

The best feeling in the world that you can give to yourself (and anyone you know):

___ ___ ___ ___
N1 K2 P1 E3

You no longer have to feel this silly way because of a stupid self-harming episode:

___ ___ ___ ___ ___ ___ H
E2 G1 G3 A3 O1 C1 xx

What you should be looking at before you buy any food or personal car product?

_ _ _ _ _ _ _ _ _ _ _

A1 O2 E1 C3 D3 H1 D2 P3 J3 L2 C1

When you hit anxious or distressing moments in life you will have this kind of willing coping mechanism:

_ _ _ _ _ A _ _ _

B1 G2 N1 F2 C3 D1 O2 O3 P3

The feeling you get when you can boast about resisting the urge to self-harm:

_ _ _ _ _

L3 C3 A1 H1 A2

After you self-harmed, you watched your skin do this many times. No more.

B _ _ _ _

xx N1 M3 F2 K3

One of the biggest elements you get back when you don't waste it on self-harm (tick tock!):

_ _ _ _

L1 D2 J2 D3

Your cells have a chance to renew and as a result your skin might look:

_ _ U _ _ _ _

K1 N2 xx J3 E1 P3 C3

The certain and trusted feeling you will have when you no longer have to hide your face:

_ _ _ _ _ _ _ _ _ _

O3 M1 J3 H2 M2 F3 A2 O2 O3 I2

The title of the second section in this Workbook

A _ A _ _ _ _ _

B2 J3 N3 C2 K1 C1 M2 C1

What you ____ on expands.

_ _ _ U _

B3 G2 O3 xx C1

CREATE MY SELF-PORTRAIT

You've come a long way. Do not look back at your first self-portrait. Start fresh with where you are at now. Draw the portrait of who you are becoming based on the way you feel or see yourself after completing many of the exercises in this book. Remember, there are no right or wrong ways to be creative. Just draw!

MEDITATION - VISIONING

Between the SPOM main text and this Workbook, you have access to a ton of more information that you were not privy to before. Consider how you have more control to change your life now. *Now* I want you to jump straight out of the "now" and into the future! Projecting a positive future can help you cement your acceptance of a better life for yourself and keep you motivated. And when you are having a tough time being in the present moment, going into a positive future meditation, is a whole lot better than staying in a worry-anxiety state of mind.

Find a nice quiet spot. Take a moment to sit and get into a meditative state of mind. Think about your life one year from now. Imagine where you will be and how you will be living. Just imagine a blissful future moment in time. It does not have to be anything too drastic, but you will feel differently. You have been eating much better, crying and releasing old resentments (and releasing newer ones closer to the moment they happen), and forgiving a lot more.

What kind of day is it? Is it sunny or cloudy? Do you wear less makeup? So does the surface of your skin feel lighter? And can you feel the sun or the wind or mist on your cheeks? What kinds of sounds do you hear? Are they happy peaceful blissful sounds? Children laughing? Ocean waves crashing? Leaves rustling? Do you notice any particular smells? You have stopped using so many petrochemical-perfumed products, so now what do you smell? Do you smell some nice essential oil that you put on or perhaps nothing on yourself, just nature smells around you? Make sure you check in with all of your senses.

Knowing that you no longer harm yourself and it's been a year since you embarked on this journey, how do you feel? Do you feel satisfied? Relieved? Triumphant? How does it feel to be free of the shame and guilt that you used to carry around with you? And how do you feel about moving forward with your life? Are you excited or curious about the road ahead no longer defining yourself as a person who self-harms?

Commit this possible future to memory!

EXCORIATION DISORDER DIAGRAM

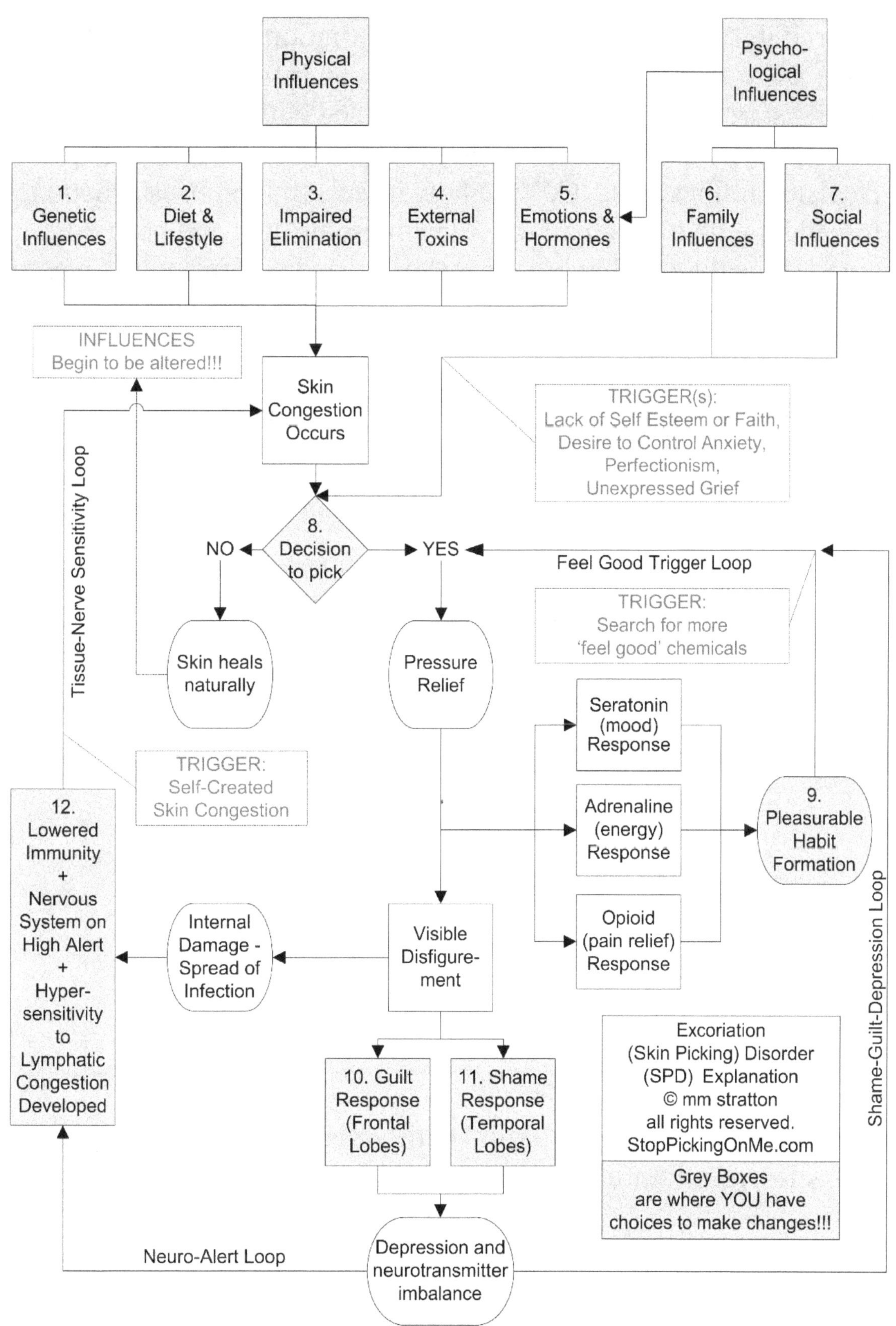

<u>Keep up the Good Work</u>

Look through the Stop Picking On Me Excoriation Disorder (SPD) Diagram. Now that you are more aware of you influencers and behaviors, start at the top of the page and trace with your finger along the lines that you used to follow. Now trace along line the lines where the Decision to Pick is: "NO." See how it feels to loop back around to the top and not go through all those troublesome step and behaviors. You are left dealing with what the rest of the world deals with: everyday normal problems!!! What a relief!

Eventually, I believe that if you follow my advice, especially about the dietary and mindfulness stuff, you will find total recovery like I have. Then the next question is what will you do with your newfound life and all of the extra time you now have, now that you're not wasting it in front of a mirror?

Action Exercise

Write down three specific actions that you will take as a result of reading the main SPOM! Text and doing the exercises in this Workbook:

1.

2.

3.

Congratulations. You are on a solid path to recovery. I wish you many blessings for your future.

Best,

Mary-Margaret (anand)

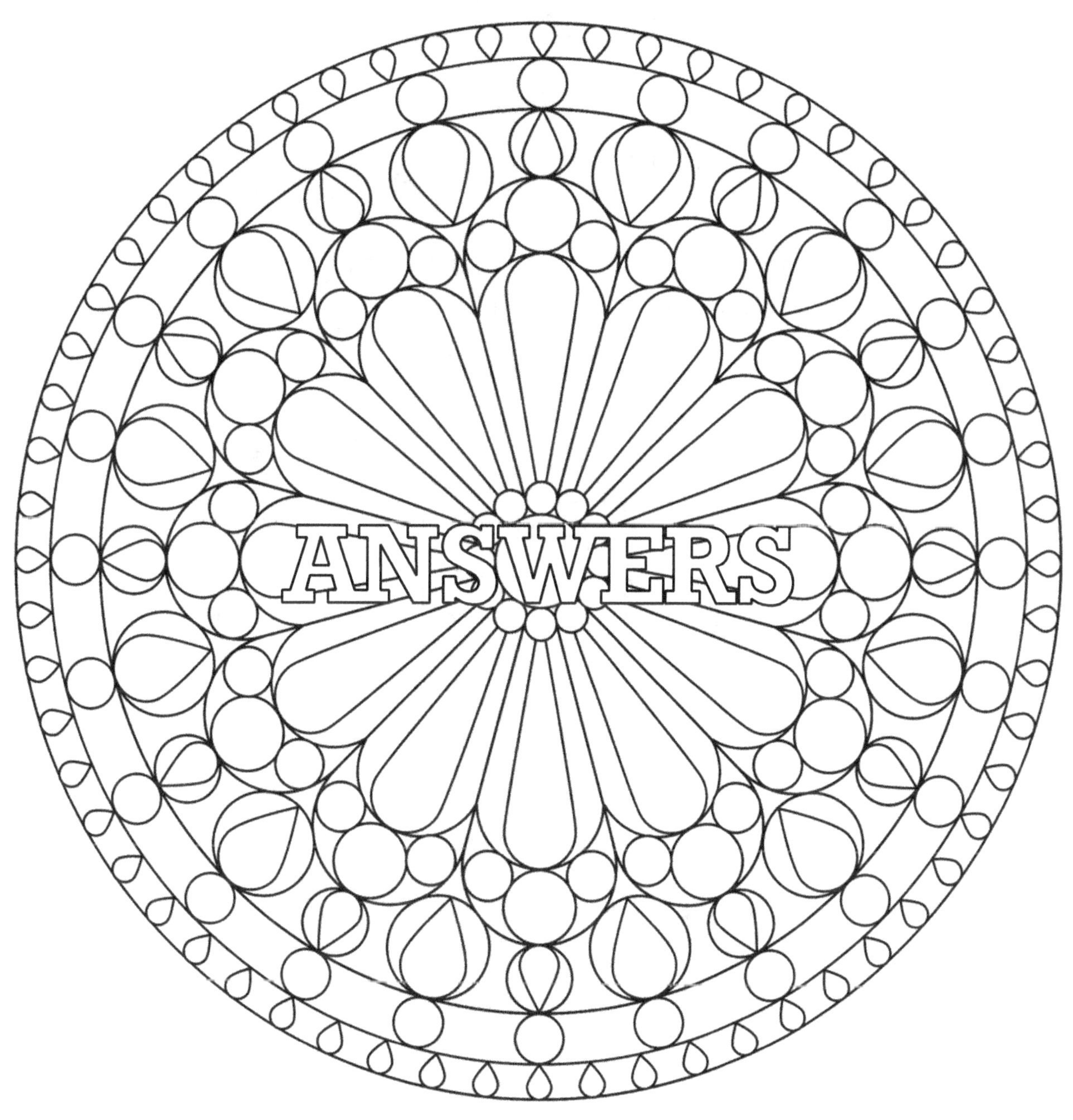

Color Me Resourceful.

Answers

Page25

B	B				S		E	L	B	A	V	O	L	
L			E		M						P			
E			A		A					A		B		
S				U	R				T		E			C
S	P	R	E	T	T	Y		I		F			A	
E						I	E		R			P		Y
D	C					N	F	E			A		P	
L		O			T		E	U		B		P	E	T
U		C	M	G	N	I	V	O	L		A		A	N
F		A		P				E	M	H			C	A
E		L			E	H	A	N	D	S	O	M	E	I
T	I	M	P	O	R	T	A	N	T				F	D
A		G	N	I	L	A	E	H					U	A
R			A	T	T	A	I	N	G	O	A	L	L	R
G					S	T	R	A	T	E	G	I	E	S

Page 49

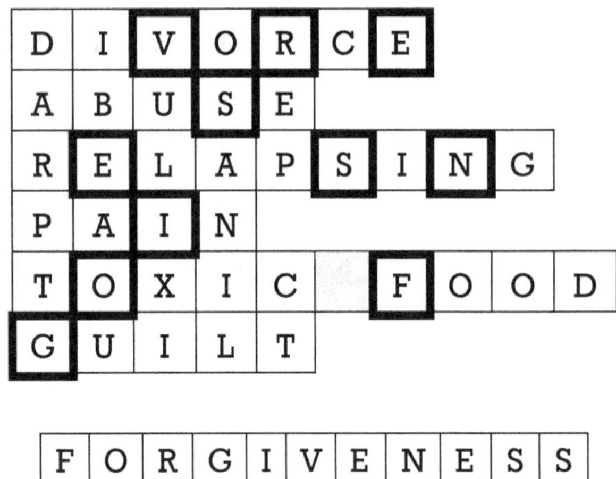

ANSWERS

Page 74

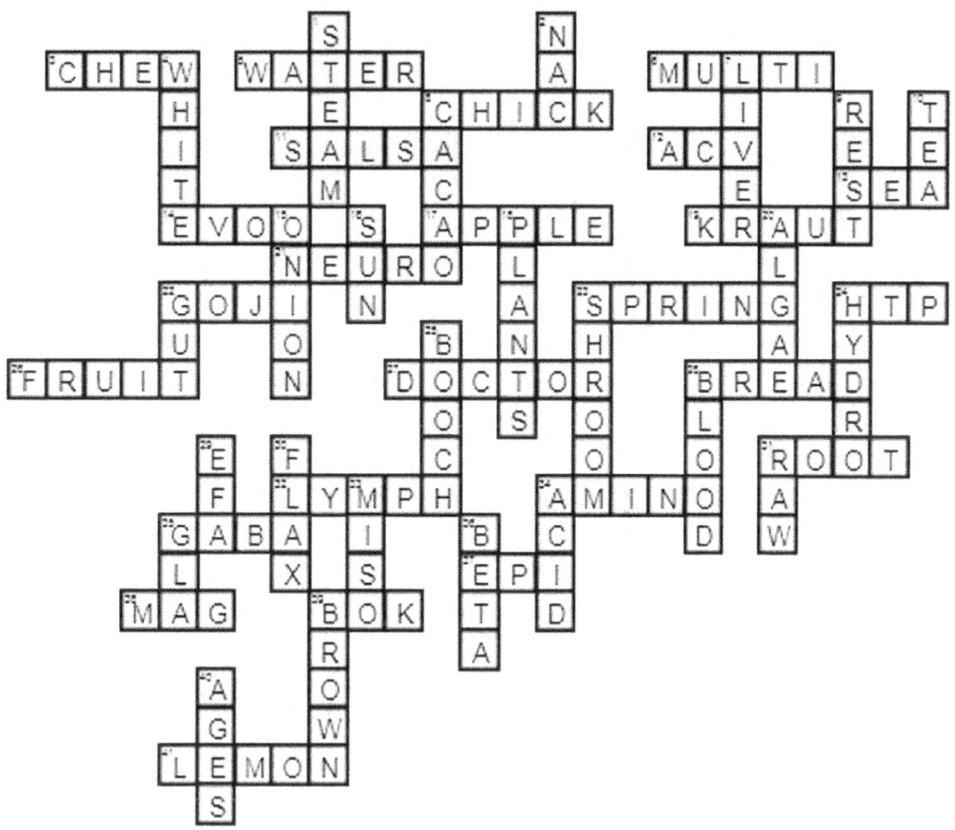

Page 78

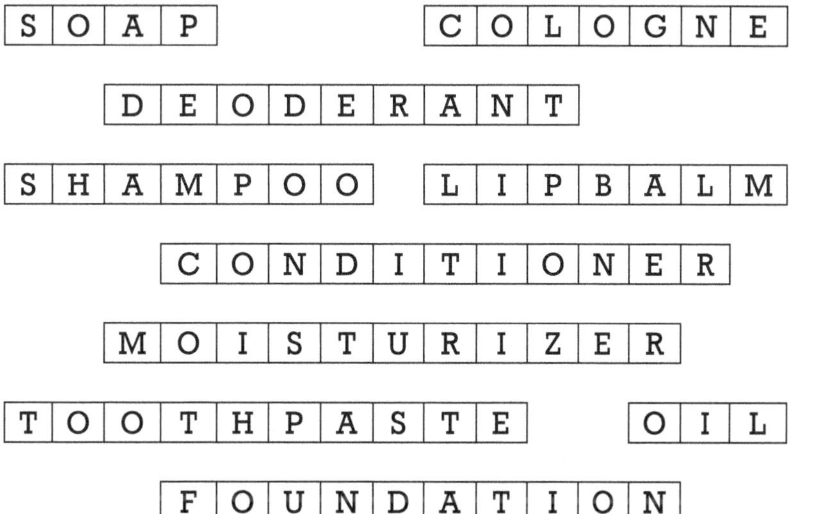

Answers

Page 89 (multiple paths will win)

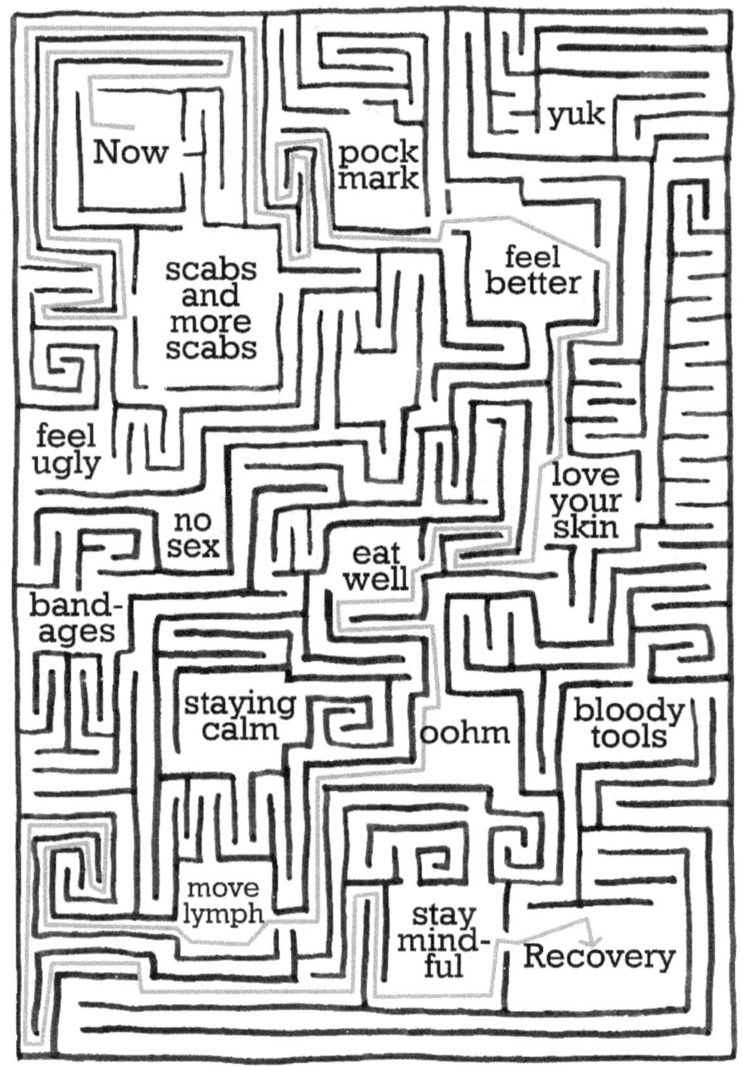

Page 123

The Phrase:
IT'S A GOOD DAY TO LIVE A LIFE OF EMOTIONAL FREEDOM
AND PEACE

The Words:
FREEDOM – LOVE – FOOLISH – INGREDIENTS – TOLERANCE
PRIDE – BLEED – TIME – YOUNGER – CONFIDENCE
ANALYSIS – FOCUS

ABOUT THE AUTHOR

Mary-Margaret (anand sahaja) Stratton is a Renaissance woman whose expertise spans a number of subjects: published poet, accomplished musical composer, prolific author, lay architect, instruction designer, painter, sculptor, festival producer, educator, and Award-Winning Creative Art Director. She has degrees in Marketing, and Design from UCLA. Anand was born and raised in the City of Angels and is currently on the Advisory Board for *Valley Relics Museum*. **She forgot to mention in her SPOM! main text biography that many years of her career were dedicated to Corporate Training using "Accelerated Learning Techniques" like the kinds you'll find in this workbook!**

Her lifelong interest in esoteric spirituality led her to write an introductory books on Paganism called ***the Good Wiccan Guides***. In 2011 anand was ordained by a Bishop of *the Essene School*. Anand received Certification as a Raw Food Nutritionist from the *Body Mind Institute and* edited a raw nutrition compendium, ***Dominant Heath***. And she was pleased to contribute ghost writing, recipes, photos and illustrations, for the raw food recipe book, ***Eat Like Eve***.

Anand is a social media evangelist and ran two online support communities for over fifteen years, including one for women with Skin Picking Disorder. She is a former Marketing Chair for the *Alliance for Addiction Solutions and* recently completed the book ***Kiss Addiction Goodbye – the Twelve Step Diet to Aid Recovery and Help Heal Addictive or Compulsive Behaviors.***

Anand has been successfully married for over twenty five years. She and her husband write music, make silly movies, travel, teach raw chocolate classes, plant urban gardens, and have been dedicated Historic Preservationists who have restored multiple Modern homes, and were recipients of the Las Vegas *MUDA, Mayor's Urban Design Award*. When not pursuing other eclectic endeavors, she likes to dance, sing, garden and watch movies with happy endings.